RECLAIM YOUR LIFE FROM IBS

A Scientifically Proven Plan for
Relief without Restrictive Diets

RECLAIM YOUR LIFE FROM
IBS

MELISSA G. HUNT, PhD

Foreword by AARON T. BECK, MD

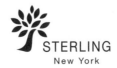

STERLING
New York

STERLING
New York

An Imprint of Sterling Publishing
1166 Avenue of the Americas
New York, NY 10036

ISBN 978-1-4549-1887-5

Distributed in Canada by Sterling Publishing Co., Inc.
c/o Canadian Manda Group, 664 Annette Street
Toronto, Ontario, Canada M6S 2C8
Distributed in the United Kingdom by GMC Distribution Services
Castle Place, 166 High Street, Lewes, East Sussex, England BN7 1XU
Distributed in Australia by Capricorn Link (Australia) Pty. Ltd.
P.O. Box 704, Windsor, NSW 2756, Australia

For information about custom editions, special sales, and premium and corporate purchases, please
contact Sterling Special Sales at 800-805-5489 or specialsales@sterlingpublishing.com.

Manufactured in Canada

2 4 6 8 10 9 7 5 3 1

www.sterlingpublishing.com

I am extraordinarily grateful to the many patients I have worked with over the last twenty-five years. Their courage, hope, resilience, insight, and willingness to take risks in therapy never fail to inspire me. This book is dedicated to them.

CONTENTS

ABOUT THE AUTHOR
AND THIS BOOK

My name is Melissa G. Hunt and I'm a licensed clinical psychologist, specializing in cognitive-behavioral therapy. I serve as the associate director of clinical training in the Department of Psychology at the University of Pennsylvania. I am very fortunate to have a career in which I can combine teaching, supervising young clinicians, doing research, and seeing patients. Each aspect of my professional life informs the others. I know that seeing patients makes me a better scientist, and doing research makes me a more effective therapist. I am always amazed that distressed people entrust me with their personal stories and are willing to share their pain in hopes that they may be able to feel better and to live more productive, rich, and joyful lives. I am always thrilled when basic and applied science can be brought to bear to improve our treatments and help people feel better.

This workbook grew directly out of my experiences working with a number of patients with gut problems in my private practice. In fact, it was my work with patients with various GI issues that led to my developing and testing the treatment in this book. This workbook is also the result of the many years I have spent engaged in the study and investigation of cognitive-behavioral therapy (CBT) approaches to understanding depression, anxiety, and life stress. CBT is a very problem-focused, practical approach to managing life's difficulties. It is also strongly grounded in science. That means the interventions you see here grew out of basic scientific principles. It *also* means that CBT has been tested in hundreds of scientific studies. Each study that is done helps us determine whether or not a treatment approach is helpful to people with a particular problem. Treatment studies also help us understand *how* and *why* a particular set of interventions may be helpful. I'm very proud of the fact that I tested *this workbook* in a randomized, controlled trial (the gold standard in science for showing that a treatment actually works), and that the people who completed it typically experienced a lot of relief. In the trial, people completed the book in six weeks. We had them read Chapters 1, 2, and 3 the first week, Chapter 4 the second week, Chapter 5 the third week, Chapter 6 the fourth week, Chapter 7 the fifth week, and Chapters 8 and 9 the sixth week. This seemed to give people enough time to read and do the exercises and set a good pace for learning and practicing the various skills. Since we know that worked well, I suggest you try to do the same.

I'm thrilled to be able to make this treatment available to a broader audience. As a therapist, for me there is no greater satisfaction than helping people. I hope this book helps you.

FOREWORD

It has been nearly forty years since I published *Cognitive Therapy and the Emotional Disorders*, and I am delighted that practitioners of cognitive-behavioral therapy continue to expand the range of disorders it can be applied to. Cognitive-behavioral therapy, or CBT, was a revolutionary approach in its day. Although I had been trained in psychoanalysis, I found that focusing on my patients' beliefs and thoughts in the here and now often led to an almost immediate lessening of symptoms. Unlike earlier models of personality and psychopathology, which assumed that people were essentially irrational and motivated to be self-destructive, cognitive therapy started with the assumption that people were basically rational and were motivated to be healthy, safe, and well. Unfortunately, sometimes people developed beliefs that were incorrect or experienced systematic bias in the way they interpreted experiences. That led them to engage in behaviors that didn't serve them well and left them far more distressed and impaired than they needed to be. Cognitive therapy, together with advances in learning theory and behavior therapy, soon became a full-fledged system of psychotherapy. CBT is inherently optimistic, respectful, and collaborative. In addition, there are two very important components to CBT that I think this book exemplifies. First, therapeutic interventions need to be grounded in a scientific understanding of what is causing people to experience distress and impairment. That is, the principles guiding therapy need to be based on scientific theory, and the therapeutic strategies need to follow naturally from those principles. Second, solid empirical findings based on randomized, controlled trials are necessary to support the efficacy of the approach—that is, to prove that it is actually helpful to people. This book is based on all of these fundamental principles.

Since my early work in the field developing cognitive therapy for depression, CBT has been applied successfully to a wide array of psychological and medical disorders, including a range of anxiety disorders, obsessive-compulsive disorder, post-traumatic stress disorder, borderline personality disorder, and medical disorders such as chronic pain, hypertension, and chronic fatigue syndrome. Irritable bowel syndrome is a chronic condition that causes a great deal of human suffering, pain, lost productivity, and high medical costs. Traditional medical management doesn't do much to relieve symptoms or improve quality of life for patients with IBS. Professionally delivered CBT, however, works quite well, which we know from numerous clinical trials. Unfortunately, finding a trained and certified cognitive therapist to work with is simply not possible for many patients with IBS. That is why I am so pleased that Dr. Melissa Hunt has written this book. A highly qualified and experienced cognitive-behavioral therapist, researcher, supervisor, and fellow of the Academy of Cognitive Therapy, she has taken the core scientific principles and strategies that comprise CBT, applied them specifically to the experience of IBS, and made it all available to any IBS patient who wants access to this excellent treatment approach. Moreover, she has tested the efficacy of this very book in a randomized, controlled trial, and found solid empirical evidence that it works.

The purpose of Dr. Melissa Hunt's book is to make quality cognitive-behavioral therapy available to all of those suffering from IBS who want to improve their quality of life, and she has succeeded admirably in this mission.

Aaron T. Beck, MD
University Professor of Psychiatry
University of Pennsylvania School of Medicine

RECLAIM YOUR LIFE FROM IBS

Chapter One

DO I HAVE IBS?

Monica is a twenty-eight-year-old woman who works as an account representative at a midsized public relations firm. Bright, hardworking, creative, and driven, she is considered a rising star by her manager. But Monica has an awful, embarrassing problem that she works hard to keep secret from her coworkers and clients. She suffers from frequent bouts of diarrhea.

When the urge to defecate comes on her suddenly and powerfully, she is never sure she'll make it to the bathroom in time. During these attacks, it feels like a red-hot hand has reached into her gut, grabbed her intestines, and tied them into knots. The burning, cramping pain is so agonizing it can bring tears to her eyes. The urgency is so intense, she fears losing control of her bowels altogether and soiling herself. The only thing that brings relief from the pain is defecating. It's manageable when it happens at home and she can simply run to the bathroom. But she fears having an attack when she is on the road or when she is trapped in a meeting at work.

She knows stress makes it worse. There was the time she was scheduled to present a new campaign concept to an important client, and she spent the entire morning at home on and off the toilet. She almost called in sick but ended up making it to the meeting with only minutes to spare.

She also knows some foods make it worse—raw vegetables, coffee, and very greasy food seem to trigger attacks. On the other hand, oatmeal and bananas seem to calm her gut.

She has tried a range of remedies, dietary changes, and over-the-counter medications. She stopped drinking milk and switched to soy milk. Unfortunately, her cramping and diarrhea symptoms didn't change, though she did seem to get more gas. Her doctor recommended eating more fiber, but she found that adding bran cereal made her symptoms worse. Then she tried eliminating gluten, but the restrictive diet was hard to maintain and it didn't seem to make a difference to her symptoms anyway. Imodium® gives her some relief and she'll pop one or two pills on the morning of a particularly busy or difficult day at work. Recently, she has started to carry Lomotil® in her purse for emergencies and will take it if she feels the twinges or spasms that often herald an attack. However, this sometimes leads to several days of no bowel movements at all. While this can be a relief for a few days, the end result of this is often constipation and bloating. When she eventually feels the urge to go again, she often has to strain and push. She's developed some painful, itchy hemorrhoids as a result, which sometimes bleed a bit when she defecates.

All in all, Monica is sick of the constant merry-go-round of diarrhea and constipation, sick of the pain and fear of being too far from a bathroom, and desperate for some relief.

If Monica's story sounds all too familiar to you, you may have IBS. Irritable bowel syndrome is a condition in which people experience recurrent abdominal pain or discomfort, along with a change in *how often* they defecate and/or a change in the *form* of the stool itself. For most people, the pain or discomfort is relieved by defecation.

As you may know, IBS is often hard to diagnose. There are two reasons for this. First, two of the main symptoms of IBS (abdominal pain and diarrhea) are common to a number of other disorders as well. The second reason IBS may be hard to diagnose is that there are no tests for it. You can't see it on an x-ray, a CT scan, or an MRI. You can't detect it in blood work. Your doctor wouldn't be able to see inflammation or polyps (little abnormal, fleshy growths) or lesions if he or she did a colonoscopy or an endoscopy. In fact, your bowels, or intestines, will *appear* perfectly normal across a range of diagnostic exams and tests. Nevertheless, they don't seem to work, or function, in a way that is smooth, painless, and efficient—that is to say, normally. Because the only problem we can identify for sure is that the GI system is not *functioning* normally, IBS is classed as a *functional gastrointestinal disorder*. This distinguishes IBS from other problems, such as the *inflammatory bowel diseases (IBDs)*, in which doctors can observe pathological changes in the tissues of the intestines.

This makes IBS, to some extent, a diagnosis of exclusion. That is, to be positive that your problem is IBS, and not something else, doctors need to rule out other reasonable causes of your symptoms. In some cases this can be done by simply reviewing your symptoms with you in detail. The doctor will need to know when your symptoms started, whether the symptoms come and go, where the pain is, what it feels like, and so on. The doctor will want to do an abdominal exam in which he or she will palpate, or feel, your abdomen with his or her hands. The doctor will also want to do some basic blood work to rule out things like infection and anemia. If the doctor is still not sure whether you have IBS or some other medical condition, the doctor may order more extensive tests, including more blood work (to check for celiac disease), a breath test (to check for lactose intolerance), imaging studies like x-rays or CT scans (to check for diverticulitis), a magnetic resonance enterography (MRE) (to check for strictures or scarring), a fecal occult blood test (to check for blood in your stool), and a fecal calprotectin test (to check for inflammation). If you have any "alarm" symptoms (e.g., fever, pain that wakes you up at night, elevated inflammatory markers in your blood work, blood or inflammatory markers in your stool), your doctor may order a colonoscopy, a sigmoidoscopy, or an endoscopy, in which the doctor can actually take a look at parts of the intestines and even take small tissue samples, or biopsies. While these tests may seem time-consuming, invasive, and uncomfortable, it's very important to be sure you've ruled out the alternative diagnoses before concluding with certainty that you have IBS. Many of these other disorders have serious complications that can result in long-term damage to your body if they're not treated appropriately. So the first step in fixing your GI problems is being sure you've got the right diagnosis. If all these other tests come back negative, then you almost certainly have IBS.

To complicate matters a bit more, it is actually possible to develop IBS *in addition to* or *shortly after* experiencing some other condition. For example, it is not uncommon for people to develop what is called post-infectious IBS. This means that the person had a serious GI infection of some kind—food poisoning, a bad stomach virus, or a C-difficile (Clostridium difficile, often referred to as C-diff) bacterial infection. In these cases there is a clear infectious agent—a bacteria or a virus that causes acute symptoms. But *after* the infection resolves, the person continues to experience significant GI symptoms, including abdominal pain and diarrhea. The same is true for the inflammatory bowel diseases like Crohn's and ulcerative colitis. People may technically be in remission from their IBD—with no evidence of inflammation in the tissues of the intestine—but may continue experiencing serious GI symptoms because they have developed secondary IBS. (See page 10 for more information on inflammatory bowel diseases and IBS.)

But just because we don't have a positive test for IBS doesn't mean it isn't a real disorder. IBS *is* a real and treatable condition in its own right. It is definitely *not* "all in your head." Your gut really isn't working right, even if we don't know exactly why. The Rome Foundation, an independent, not-for-profit organization dedicated to research and education about functional gastrointestinal disorders, has published the following criteria for diagnosing irritable bowel syndrome.

ROME III DIAGNOSTIC CRITERIA FOR
FUNCTIONAL GASTROINTESTINAL DISORDERS

Irritable Bowel Syndrome

*Diagnostic Criteria**

Recurrent abdominal pain or discomfort (an uncomfortable sensation not described as pain) at least three days a month in the last three months associated with *two or more* of the following:

1. Improvement with defecation.
2. Onset associated with a change in frequency of stool.
3. Onset associated with a change in form (appearance) of stool.

If you're a woman, the pain does not occur only during your menstrual cycle.

Some people with IBS experience mostly diarrhea (diarrhea-predominant IBS) and some people experience mostly constipation (constipation-predominant IBS), but many people with IBS actually have both hard and loose stools over periods of hours, days, or weeks (mixed-type IBS). Other kinds of discomfort are also associated with IBS, including:

- Feeling "gassy" or "bloated" (which sometimes results in flatulence or farting).
- Feeling a *sudden urge* to have a bowel movement.
- Straining during defecation.

* Criteria fulfilled for the last three months with symptom onset at least six months prior to diagnosis.

- Feeling as if you "can't get it all out."

- Having fewer than three bowel movements a week.

- Having more than three bowel movements a day.

The funny thing about these symptoms is that lots of people who *don't* have IBS (or any other GI disorder) experience these symptoms, too, at least sometimes. That is, there's a big range of what people consider "normal" in their bowel habits. What seems to distinguish people who have IBS from people who don't is partly the *severity* and *frequency* of GI symptoms. But it's also important to take into account how *distressing* the symptoms are to you, and how much you feel you are *impaired* by the symptoms as you try to go about your normal life.

Many physicians now feel comfortable diagnosing IBS on the basis of a review of symptoms, an abdominal exam in which the doctor palpates, or feels, your abdomen, and a few simple medical tests, such as blood work to rule out infection and anemia. If you don't have any "alarm" symptoms (like fever, blood or inflammatory markers in your stool, inflammatory markers in your blood, anemia or other nutritional deficiencies, or abdominal pain that awakens you at night), current medical practice is to avoid further invasive diagnostic testing, because it is statistically unlikely that you will have a more serious condition. However, it is important to keep in mind that many medical conditions, some of which are easy to manage *if you know you have them*, share symptoms with IBS. In particular, it is probably worth being tested for *lactose intolerance* and *celiac disease*. If you *do* have IBS, the treatment and skills outlined in this workbook should be very helpful to you. If you have one of these other conditions, you need to follow up with a gastroenterologist. That doesn't mean these skills won't help—they probably will, especially if you have secondary IBS—but you need to be sure the medical condition is also being appropriately managed.

OTHER CONDITIONS THAT MAY SHARE SYMPTOMS WITH IBS

Diarrhea and abdominal pain, in particular, can occur in a range of gastrointestinal diseases and conditions, so it is very important to consult with your physician to be confident that you have ruled them out. Conditions that share symptoms with IBS fall into several basic categories. These include the inflammatory bowel diseases, genuine intolerance of certain foods, diverticulitis, cancer (which is extremely rare), and intestinal parasites.

Inflammatory Bowel Diseases

Crohn's Disease
Crohn's disease is an inflammatory bowel disease that can cause abdominal pain and diarrhea. Crohn's disease can also cause rectal bleeding, weight loss, ulcers in the intestines, arthritis, skin problems, and fever. Sometimes the bleeding is so serious that it leads to anemia, and people may develop malnutrition as the inflammation of the lining of the intestines worsens. Crohn's disease can also cause ulcers or sores in other parts of the body, including the mouth, the throat, and the esophagus. Sometimes the intestines actually become blocked by thickened scar tissue (adhesions and strictures) that are the result of long-term inflammation. Crohn's disease is an autoimmune disorder in which the body's immune system starts to attack both helpful (symbiotic) bacteria, which normally live in the gut, and gut tissue itself. This chronic inflammatory response causes damage to the digestive tract, which can result in ulcers, thickened scar tissue, tears, bleeding, and malnutrition, including anemia secondary to blood loss and more general nutritional deficits due to malabsorption of food.

To diagnose Crohn's disease, your doctor will check for a number of things. In a blood test, many people with Crohn's will show signs of anemia, which can suggest that the ulcers in the intestines are causing bleeding. Because Crohn's disease is an inflammatory process, the blood test will often show inflammatory markers, sometimes including a high white blood cell count. In addition to blood work, the doctor will probably also ask you to take stool samples for several days, and will check those samples for blood (called a fecal occult blood test) and for a special marker called fecal calprotectin, which suggests that there is inflammation in the tissues of the intestines.

Your doctor will probably also want to get a good look at your intestines. There are a number of ways to do this. In an upper GI series, you will need to drink barium, a slightly sweet, chalky white liquid that coats the lining of the small intestine, making it easier to see what's going on. After drinking the barium, you will have x-rays or a CT scan taken. The barium looks white in the images and shows spots where there may be inflammation or other abnormalities in the small intestine. In a lower GI series, you will have to take barium in the form of an enema, which will be administered by the doctor. Then x-rays or CT scans are taken of your large intestines, including the colon and rectum. Another kind of imaging study is a magnetic resonance enterography, or MRE. In an MRE, you still have to drink a contrast fluid (like the barium). Then you get an IV and have MRE images taken. This test is more sensitive than CT scans, and can get images in real time. This lets it distinguish between the strictures seen in IBDs and normal peristalsis (or contractions) of the intestines.

Another way to get a look at different parts of your intestines is for the doctor to do an actual visual exam by performing either a sigmoidoscopy or a colonoscopy. In both of these procedures, the doctor inserts a flexible, lighted tube into the anus and up through part of the large intestine. Flexible sigmoidoscopy lets the doctor see only the last third of the large intestine (the sigmoid colon). Colonoscopy allows the doctor to see the *entire* large intestine or colon, and *sometimes* the ileum (the lowest part of the small intestine), so it's usually the better procedure, although it does take a bit more time to prepare for, and it usually requires sedation or anesthesia. In both cases, the scope transmits images of the lining of the intestine to a computer or video monitor. In an upper endoscopy, the doctor will be able to look at the esophagus, the stomach, and the upper part of the small intestine. None of these procedures allow the doctor to look at the middle part of the small intestine, and it can be difficult to see the ileum during a colonoscopy.

The best way to visualize the entire small intestine is with a capsule endoscopy. In this amazing procedure, you swallow a tiny camera that is safely inside a capsule no bigger than the average vitamin pill. As it travels through the GI tract, it transmits multiple pictures to a small receiver worn on a belt. The capsule is disposable and passes out of your system with a bowel movement. (You don't have to worry about trying to retrieve it!) The advantage of this is that it lets your doctor see the entire small intestine, which is where Crohn's often has its effects. All these procedures allow the doctor to actually *see* if there is any inflammation, ulcers, or bleeding. Both colonoscopy and sigmoidoscopy also allow the doctor to remove any polyps or other growths and to take very small samples of tissue or biopsies, which can then be looked at carefully under a microscope.

Ulcerative Colitus

Ulcerative colitis is the other main inflammatory bowel disease. UC, like Crohn's disease, can also cause inflammation and ulcers in the lining of the rectum and colon, but, unlike Crohn's disease, the inflammation occurs only in the top layer of the lining of the large intestine. Ulcers can form where inflammation has killed the cells that usually line the colon. Like Crohn's disease, this can often result in intestinal bleeding, leading to anemia and bloody stools. Like IBS and Crohn's, the most common symptoms of ulcerative colitis are abdominal pain or cramps and frequent diarrhea. Other complications include anemia, weight loss, loss of appetite, fever, skin lesions, joint pain, and rectal bleeding. Like Crohn's disease, UC is thought to result from a disorder of the immune system.

UC is diagnosed in much the same way Crohn's disease is, with sigmoid-oscopy or colonoscopy. Blood tests may show anemia and a high white blood cell count or other inflammatory markers. A stool sample may reveal blood or elevated fecal calprotectin. A lower GI series may well show evidence of inflammation or ulcers. The best way of diagnosing UC is with a colonoscopy or sigmoidoscopy. Because UC differs from Crohn's disease in how deep the inflammation goes in the intestinal wall, the doctor will need to take tissue samples for microscopic analysis to make a definitive diagnosis.

Can I Have Both IBD and IBS?

For most people who are ultimately diagnosed with an inflammatory bowel disease, the journey to diagnosis is long and harrowing. Many patients have been through the proverbial medical wringer—seeing an average of five different doctors, undergoing an average of eight or nine diagnostic tests, and spending more than a year feeling very ill (with almost half of patients being hospitalized at least once) before they finally get a positive diagnosis. Just hearing that someone has *finally* figured out what's wrong with you may actually be a relief. In fact, IBD patients are sometimes *misdiagnosed* with IBS for *years* before someone finally figures out what's really going on.

So what do you make of it if a doctor tells you that your IBD is in remission, but you are still having GI symptoms because *now* you have IBS!? Is that even possible!? Unfortunately, it is. In fact, some studies suggest that about *half* of IBD patients will experience IBS-like symptoms when the IBD itself is in remission. Put another way, IBD patients are about three times as likely to develop IBS as someone in the general population. This may seem horribly unfair. But the good news is that if this is you, then the treatment in the rest of this book should help a lot.

Celiac Disease

Celiac disease is an autoimmune disorder in which the body is unable to break down gluten, one of the major proteins in wheat, rye, and barley.

When people with celiac disease eat foods containing gluten (like bread and pasta), their immune system treats the gluten as a foreign invader and mounts a huge defensive response. Unfortunately, this results in damage to the wall of the small intestine. The small intestine is lined with villi—tiny, fingerlike projections that coat the lining of the small intestine and dramatically increase the surface area available for absorbing nutrients from food. In celiac disease, the villi are damaged or even destroyed. The most common symptoms of celiac disease are—you guessed it—abdominal pain and diarrhea (and sometimes constipation), although the stools in celiac disease are usually pale in color. The second most common symptom in adults is anemia, due to malabsorption of nutrients. Like the inflammatory bowel diseases, celiac disease can also manifest itself in other parts of the body, leading to fatigue, joint pain, arthritis, canker sores in the mouth, or an itchy rash on the skin. People with celiac disease usually find that their symptoms get worse after eating certain foods—but so do people with IBS. You can see why celiac disease, the inflammatory bowel diseases, and IBS can be very difficult to distinguish from one another on the basis of symptoms alone.

To make a positive diagnosis of celiac disease, the doctor will start with bloodwork. Anemia (especially if it doesn't resolve quickly with iron supplements) is a clue that, whatever is going on, it is probably *not* IBS. One very specific test for celiac disease is to look for certain antibodies in the blood. It is very important to continue eating a diet that contains gluten for approximately six weeks before the test. If you are already on a gluten-free diet, the tests will come back negative, even if you really do have celiac disease. Celiac disease is partly genetic, and there is actually a genetic test available to see if you carry the genes for it. If you don't, then you *can't* have celiac disease. If you *do* carry the genes, then you *might* have celiac disease.

If your symptoms and blood work (and possibly genetic testing) are consistent with celiac disease, your doctor will probably want to do an endoscopy, in which a flexible, thin tube is inserted through the mouth and stomach to reach the small intestine. Celiac disease affects the villi in the small intestine. During an endoscopy, the doctor will be able to see the lining of the small intestine and will be able to take tissue samples to confirm whether the villi have been damaged.

While celiac disease is sometimes present from childhood, it can be triggered in adulthood by a variety of environmental and physical stressors, including surgery, pregnancy, viral infection, or even severe emotional stress. So just because you never had trouble with gluten-containing foods earlier in life doesn't necessarily mean you don't have celiac disease now. Celiac disease can be managed entirely with dietary changes—you have to stop eating gluten. The good news is that a gluten-free diet will stop the damage and allow your intestines to heal. Unfortunately, a truly gluten-free diet is tricky to maintain. There is "hidden" gluten in a lot of prepared and restaurant foods. But if you educate yourself about it and commit to it, a gluten-free diet can solve your GI symptoms.

On the other hand, if you *don't* have celiac disease, it probably makes no sense at all to avoid gluten. Going "gluten free" is a popular fad right now, and there are new (and very expensive) products showing up on the gluten-free shelves every day. This has been a moneymaking, marketing bonanza for industrial food companies—replacing "fat free" and "sugar free" as a way to appeal to health-conscious but naive consumers. For people with true celiac, the availability of gluten-free products has been an incredible blessing. In fact, certain gluten-free products (like special breads and pastas) are tax deductible for people with celiac disease because they are a medical necessity. For most people, however, avoiding gluten makes no sense and will not have an impact on GI functioning or overall health. Most human beings have no difficulty digesting this protein. Indeed, barley, wheat, and rye have been important staple foods for a significant proportion of the human population for millennia. Limiting your calories from refined carbohydrates like white bread and pasta may be good for your waistline, but eating a gluten-free diet is totally unnecessary for most of us. That said, if you *do* have celiac disease, you really *must* avoid gluten or you risk long-term pain, malabsorption, nutritional deficiencies, and poor health. So it is definitely worth being tested for celiac disease with a blood test.

Lactose Intolerance

Another possible cause of GI symptoms is lactose intolerance. Lactose intolerance occurs when the small intestine does not produce the enzyme lactase, which breaks down the sugar lactose that is found in all kinds of milk. What are the symptoms of lactose intolerance? Abdominal pain, gas, bloating, and diarrhea, of course!

Interestingly, all human beings produce the lactase enzyme during the first few years of life, because lactose is found in human breast milk and is necessary for early development. In many people of the world (especially Asians, Southeast Asians, Native Americans, and some Africans), lactase production stops around age two—the time that toddlers would typically be weaned. Interestingly, traditional Asian and Native American cuisines typically contain no milk products, consistent with the fact that folks from those ethnic backgrounds do indeed tend to be lactose-intolerant. People in those cultures found ways to combine legumes (beans or soybeans) with grains (corn, rice, or wheat) to make complete proteins and provide full nutrition.

In many other human populations, however, primarily people from pastoral cultures that developed cow, sheep, and goat herding early on (including many African, most Indian, and most European and Middle Eastern peoples), a genetic mutation occurred that kept the lactase production gene *switched on*. You may have heard that humans shouldn't drink milk because we didn't "evolve" to, but in fact this is incorrect. The extended lactase production mutation occurred independently in different human populations at different times. It was a tremendous advantage under certain environmental circumstances, allowing the introduction of cow, goat, sheep, and even reindeer and yak milk products as major forms of dietary protein. Animal milk is a *fantastic* way to turn otherwise totally indigestible grass into a high-quality, complete, tasty, and versatile protein, so the ability to digest it was strongly selected for in those populations where it arose. This is actually *exactly* how evolution works—a spontaneous genetic mutation arises that confers survival and reproductive advantage and is therefore selected for and passed on to the next generation. So, in fact, lots of humans *did* evolve to drink milk. But not *all* humans did, so there are indeed some people who are lactose-intolerant. Because cow's milk has become such a major part of the Western diet, actually being lactose-intolerant in America or Europe can be quite problematic.

Lactose intolerance is diagnosed in several ways. First, your doctor may recommend trying an "elimination diet." Under this regimen, you stop eating all dairy products for several weeks and see if the symptoms go away. Then you reintroduce dairy products and see if the symptoms return. There are a number of problems with this approach. First of all, eliminating a whole class of foods usually means changing your diet in lots of ways—you typically increase something else or add a new food entirely (e.g., soy milk or almond milk). You might be reducing the amount of overall fat in your diet (no more ice cream or cheese, after all). You're probably also paying a lot more attention to what and how you're eating—not eating out as much, cooking more carefully, and so on. So it's really hard to know if any changes in your symptoms were actually due to eliminating food *A* or to introducing or increasing food(s) *B*, *C*, or *D*. Another reason elimination diets are problematic is that when you suddenly stop eating a certain type of food, the helpful, symbiotic bacteria that normally live in your gut and help digest that food may die off. When you reintroduce the food, you may feel symptomatic because you've thrown off your microbiome. So elimination diets are *not* a good way to figure out if a food is causing you problems and are pretty nonspecific from a diagnostic perspective.

A much *better* test is the hydrogen breath test. Undigested lactose is broken down by bacteria in the gut, leading to the production of hydrogen and methane gases, which can be detected in the breath. Eventually, a simple genetic test may be used to identify individuals who are lactose-intolerant, but that is not available in routine clinical practice yet. Because the hydrogen breath test, like the celiac blood test, is not particularly invasive, it's almost certainly worth doing to rule out the possibility that your symptoms are being caused by lactose intolerance.

Diverticulosis/Diverticulitis

Diverticulosis is a condition in which the walls of the colon weaken in some spots and bulge out into little balloon-shaped sacks or pouches. It is uncommon in people under the age of forty, but about half of people over the age of sixty have at least some diverticula. When the pouches become inflamed or infected, the condition is called diverticulitis. The symptoms of diverticulitis are—wait for it—cramping pain or discomfort in the abdomen and a change in bowel habits—either diarrhea or constipation. Complications of diverticulitis may also include low-grade fever and bloody stools.

Diagnosing diverticulitis starts, as always, with a thorough medical history to review the symptoms and a physical exam, including palpating the abdomen and a rectal exam, in which the doctor inserts a gloved finger into the anus and gently probes for tenderness, blockages, or blood. The typical follow-up is a lower GI series with a barium enema and imaging using x-rays or a CT scan, or an MRI. A colonoscopy can allow the doctor to see the diverticula. But if the problem has progressed to diverticulitis (inflammation), a colonoscopy may aggravate the problem.

The main treatment for diverticulosis is to increase the amount of fiber in the diet. In fact, people who eat diets high in vegetables, fruits, and whole grains and relatively low in red and processed meats have much less chance of developing diverticulosis to begin with. Note once again the importance of accurate diagnosis. If you had celiac disease, the last thing you'd want to do would be to increase the amount of whole (wheat) grain in your diet! If you have IBS, simply increasing your fiber intake is very unlikely to be helpful and may actually make your symptoms worse. (See Chapter 8, "Diet and IBS," for dietary guidelines and suggestions for IBS.)

Colorectal Cancer

Colorectal cancer (or colon cancer) occurs when cells in the large intestine start to multiply in an out-of-control way. Usually, the tumors begin as polyps—little bumps or growths inside the lining of the large intestine. Most polyps are benign. They usually don't cause symptoms and are not dangerous. But, sometimes, polyps become cancerous over time. The symptoms of colon cancer vary and depend on the location and size of the tumor and whether the cancer has metastasized (or spread) to other parts of the body, such as the liver. If the tumor is close to the anus, there may be a change in bowel habits—either diarrhea or constipation. If the tumor begins to block the flow of stools (called a bowel obstruction), the patient may experience abdominal pain, constipation, and/or vomiting. There may also be evidence of blood in the stools. The single best way to diagnose colon cancer is with a colonoscopy. If caught early, colon cancer is usually treatable. The American Gastroenterological Association advises people who have no risk factors to be tested starting at age fifty, while people with a family history of colon cancer should have their first colonoscopy at age forty, or ten years before the age that their relative got cancer, whichever comes first. If you are struggling with GI symptoms, a colonoscopy can certainly bring peace of mind if it rules out this potentially fatal disease, but if you are under fifty and have no family history of colon cancer, it's probably not worth doing, unless your doctor suspects an inflammatory bowel disease.

Intestinal Parasites

One cause of gastrointestinal problems that many Westerners do not consider is intestinal parasites. Intestinal parasites fall into two main groups—single-celled organisms (protozoans) and parasitic worms. One common protozoan parasite is giardia. Giardiasis (the condition that results after ingesting giardia, usually by drinking contaminated water) is characterized by diarrhea, abdominal cramps or pain, bloating, passing gas, and sometimes nausea. In most cases, giardiasis resolves on its own in seven to ten days. But in some cases, it becomes chronic, leading to bouts of diarrhea that come and go and frequently alternate with constipation. Sound familiar? If there is any chance you have consumed untreated water (say, from a stream while camping or while traveling in a developing nation) or if you have been around someone who has giardia, you should ask your doctor to check your stool for parasites. There are also blood tests to identify antigens specific to the giardia parasite.

One of the most common parasitic worms is the hookworm (which is actually one of two different kinds of roundworm). Hookworms are transmitted through skin contact with contaminated feces. Dogs and cats can and do contract hookworm, and simply emptying the litter box or cleaning up the dog poop in the yard can present opportunities for transmission. Hookworms have a complicated life cycle, but they end up in the intestines of the host, where they cause abdominal pain, diarrhea, and excessive gas. Long-term infection may result in anemia as the worms themselves are feeding on the blood of the host. Hookworm can be diagnosed through a stool sample.

Intestinal parasites are generally easy to treat and are often overlooked by American physicians as a source of gastrointestinal distress (although most veterinarians routinely screen for these parasites in puppies and kittens). If you own or come into contact with dogs or cats, it's probably a good idea to have your doctor check your stool for hookworms and other possible intestinal parasites.

SO, DO YOU HAVE IBS?

If your symptoms are consistent with the Rome III criteria listed on pages 5-6, you may well have IBS. To recap, the symptoms of IBS include:

Rome III Criteria:

- Recurrent, cramping abdominal pain or discomfort that is relieved with defecation.

- A change in the frequency of defecation (usually more than three bowel movements a day, or fewer than three bowel movements a week).

- A change in the appearance or consistency of stool (either loose and watery or hard and dry).

- Your symptoms started at least six months ago and have been ongoing for at least the last three months.

- If you're a woman, the discomfort and changes in stool do not occur only during menstruation.

In addition, you may also experience the following:

- Feeling "gassy" or "bloated" or increased flatulence.

- Feeling a *sudden urge* to have a bowel movement.

- Straining during defecation.

- Feeling as if you "can't get it all out."

As noted above, some physicians feel comfortable diagnosing IBS on the basis of a review of these symptoms and an abdominal exam. But, to be sure that you and your doctor have ruled out the other possible explanations, you should, at least, have blood work, including a celiac antibody test; a hydrogen breath test to rule out lactose intolerance; a fecal occult blood test and a fecal calprotectin test; and possibly a lower or upper GI imaging study, which might be an x-ray, a CT scan, or an MRE. In some cases, your doctor may feel more confident if he or she orders a colonoscopy, an endoscopy, and/or a capsule endoscopy as well.

SUMMARY

- People with IBS do *not* typically show evidence of anemia, unless they are severely restricting their diet and have eliminated too many iron-rich foods. If that is the cause of their anemia, taking an iron supplement for a week should correct the problem. Short-term iron supplementation does not necessarily help people with active Crohn's, ulcerative colitis, or celiac disease because the anemia is caused by bleeding and/or poor absorption of nutrients, not a lack of iron in the diet.

- People with IBS also do *not* typically have high white blood cell counts or other inflammatory markers, because IBS is not due directly to infection or severe inflammation. Someone with IBS might have a high white blood cell count (and have a low-grade fever) if he or she is fighting some other, unrelated infection (like a cold or the flu). If this is the case, then retesting the blood in several weeks should show a return to normal levels. But you *might* have both IBS and an inflammatory bowel disease, such as Crohn's, if you continue to experience symptoms when the IBD is in remission and your blood and GI tissues look normal.

- People with IBS do *not* typically have elevated levels of celiac antibodies, even if they eat lots of wheat and other gluten-containing foods.

- People with IBS do *not* show lactose intolerance during a hydrogen breath test.

- People with IBS do *not* typically have blood in their stools, although hemorrhoids in the rectum and around the anus may bleed a bit and contaminate the stool sample.

- People with IBS do *not* typically show evidence of inflammation, sores, diverticula, or other damage in either the small or large intestine during imaging studies, endoscopy, or colonoscopy. Again, you may have a history of positive findings if you have an inflammatory bowel disease. But if the IBD is currently in remission (that is, you're not having an active flare) and your gut currently *looks* normal but still isn't *working* right, you may have secondary IBS.

- It *is* possible to have an inflammatory bowel disease that is in remission, and then go on to develop IBS.

- People with IBS do *not* typically have intestinal parasites.

So, if you and your doctor have ruled out all of these other explanations, you almost certainly *do* have IBS. Okay, we've got a diagnosis. Great. Now what?

SUGGESTED ACTIVITIES

1. Review your medical history with your doctor and make sure you know which diagnostic tests have been done and what the results were.

2. If you are not confident that alternative explanations have been ruled out, discuss with your doctor the possibility of follow-up testing.

3. Complete the self-report questionnaires in Appendices A, B, and C. These questionnaires will give you a sense of whether you fulfill the Rome III criteria, how severe your GI symptoms are, and how much of a negative impact IBS is having on your quality of life.

Chapter Two

WHAT'S CAUSING MY GUT SYMPTOMS?

Just because IBS is not associated with visible or testable pathology or tissue damage, does not mean that IBS is not a real condition or that the symptoms are "all in your head." The symptoms of IBS—pain, diarrhea, constipation, urgency, gas, and bloating—are all real physical symptoms, as you well know.

Most IBS experts believe that IBS is the result of a number of factors, some of which are biological, some of which are psychological, and some of which are environmental (technically called a *biopsychosocial model*). Let's take a look at how all the different pieces come together to result in the constellation of symptoms we call IBS.

THE ENTERIC NERVOUS SYSTEM

Did you know that you have a brain in your gut? Well, not really. But many gastroenterologists point out that the gut has its own nervous system that has just as many nerve cells, or neurons, as the spinal cord. The enteric nervous system consists of a number of different types of neurons, each of which do different jobs. For example, motor neurons, embedded in the muscles in the digestive tract, control motility—the smooth contractions of muscles that move food through the system at just the right speed (a process called *peristalsis*) and the mixing, squishing actions that help break food down, mix it up, expose it to digestive juices, and make it available for absorption (*segmentation contractions*). Sensory neurons do lots of different jobs, including sensing or "tasting" different chemicals in the food you have eaten (like glucose and the amino acids that make up proteins), conveying information about stretch and tension in the walls of the stomach and intestines, and also relaying the perception of pain.

One contributing factor in IBS may be that both the motor neurons and the sensory neurons in the enteric nervous system are hypersensitive or hyperreactive to certain stimuli. This means several things.

1. People with IBS are more likely to *feel* normal activity in the gut. Most people are not aware of peristalsis or segmentation contractions. They don't notice if a gas bubble moves along or pops. However, the sensory neurons in people with IBS may transmit this information more "loudly" to their brain. When this happens, it focuses their attention on their gut and seems to suggest that there might be a problem going on, even if there isn't. This is called *visceral hypersensitivity*, because people become hypersensitive to sensations in their viscera, or gut; notice them more frequently; and often start to worry about them. You may be more likely to develop visceral hypersensitivity if you have a history of GI disease like Crohn's, because paying attention to gut symptoms may have been important in monitoring and tracking your symptom severity and response to medication and other treatments.

2. The motor neurons in the colon may not always
   work smoothly or in concert with each other,
   or may work too strongly at times. This is
   called *abnormal intestinal motility.* The colon,
   or large intestine, is the last five feet (1.5 m) of
   the intestine. The main job of the colon is to
   remove just the right amount of water and salt
   from digested food waste, and then hold onto
   the waste materials until it's time to defecate.
   The speed at which food waste moves through
   the colon (technically called *transit time*), and
   therefore the amount of water that is extracted
   from the stool, is controlled by the small,
   rhythmic contractions of the muscles in the
   colon called peristalsis. The overall process of
   moving food through the colon is called *motility.*
   If food waste moves through too quickly, not
   enough water is extracted, and you get loose,
   watery stools, or diarrhea. If food waste moves
   through too slowly, you get hard, dry stools,
   or constipation. Maintaining just the right level
   of motility in the colon is a delicate balance. It
   depends on lots of things, like how much fiber
   you eat, how much water you drink, how much
   exercise you get, and the level of stress in your
   life, but ultimately you need those motor neurons
   to be firing at the right rate given everything else
   that's going on.
3. Both the sensory neurons and the motor neurons
   may start to overreact or respond too strongly to
   certain kinds of foods. A big, greasy cheeseburger
   that might leave a person without IBS feeling

slightly overfull might send a person with IBS rushing to the bathroom as the enteric nervous system reacts with all kinds of loud, mixed-up signals registering the overload of fat and rushing the barely digested burger through the system.

4. People with IBS also seem to have more sensitive or reactive pain receptors in the gut than those without IBS. These receptors scream, *"Are you trying to kill me!?"* after you eat that cheeseburger, while the receptors in a person without IBS might just murmur, "Enough already." Pain grabs our attention. It's usually a signal that something is really wrong and that we'd better do something to get ourselves out of harm's way. In fact, pain is an important way of protecting ourselves. Your hand hurts when you put it on the hot stove, and that instantly triggers a reflex to pull your hand away, sparing you a bad burn. Some people are born without the ability to sense pain (called *congenital insensitivity to pain*). This sounds like a blessing, but it's really a curse. Many of these people suffer horrible disabling or disfiguring accidents, and very few survive past age twenty-five. So pain can be an important signal and can give us information that something is wrong that has to be fixed. Like a smoke detector, pain tells us there's a fire to put out.

On the other hand, overly sensitive pain receptors are *not* providing any useful information. They are more like smoke detectors that go off every time you boil water. At best that's noisy and annoying. But what if you gathered the family together and fled the house every single time it happened? You'd spend an awful lot of time feeling panicked and frantic and not much time cooking dinner! Pain receptors in the gut are supposed to tell us when we have a serious infection or have eaten something dangerous. They are *not* supposed to overreact to basically benign foods, and they're certainly not supposed to overreact to environmental and psychological stressors.

STRESS AND THE AUTONOMIC NERVOUS SYSTEM

This would all be bad enough, but the enteric nervous system doesn't operate in a vacuum. It is also in constant communication with the rest of the *autonomic nervous system,* or ANS. The rest of the ANS is actually made up of two different, parallel sets of nerve systems that have to work together in balance with each other. Both of them directly affect the functioning of the intestinal tract and "talk" back and forth with the enteric nervous system. One is called the *parasympathetic nervous system.* The other is called the *sympathetic nervous system.*

It's easiest to think about them in terms of the processes they control. The *parasympathetic* nervous system helps us *rest and digest.* Sounds like a good thing! It's responsible for managing lots of body processes that help us feel calm and at ease. This system is active when our brain tells us that everything's going well, no emergencies need attending to, and we can devote our time and attention to eating, digesting, sleeping, and generally hanging around and feeling relaxed.

The *sympathetic* nervous system, on the other hand, helps us with *fight-or-flight-or-freeze* responses. It's responsible for managing all the body processes that make us feel keyed up, alert, and ready for action. This system is active when our brain tells us that there's something dangerous or threatening in our environment that has to be dealt with by either fighting, running away, or freezing in place.

Sympathetic nervous system activation affects the *whole body*. It leads to increases in heart rate, blood pressure, respiration (breathing faster), and muscle tension. Our brain squirts out adrenaline and cortisol, and our liver makes lots of glucose (blood sugar) available to our muscles. Sympathetic nervous system activation also leads to dumping waste and urine. In a life-threatening emergency, you can't waste resources carrying around extra weight, and you're not worried about extracting those last few nutrients, so the muscles in the bladder and colon spasm to get rid of the waste. That's why people often feel a strong urge to pee or defecate when they're very frightened.

Believe it or not, this is a *great* system to have in place if you are trying to escape from a man-eating tiger. All that activation focuses your attention sharply on the threat and gives you lots of energy and power to fight (or run!) for your life. Unfortunately, it's not really a very good system to have in place if you're dealing with family conflict, rush-hour traffic, or unpaid bills. That is, most of the "threats" we face in modern life don't require a massive and immediate physical effort to manage. But that doesn't stop your body from treating a difficult meeting with your boss or an argument with a loved one the same way our ancestors treated an encounter with a saber-toothed tiger.

This means that our body's physical response to stress isn't always very helpful. We get all juiced up and then have nowhere to go with all that activation. This is why people who are chronically stressed may experience lots of different physical symptoms, like muscle spasms (especially in the neck, shoulders, and back), headaches, chest pain, hives, heartburn, indigestion, and gut problems. For people with IBS, the main symptom of sympathetic nervous system activation is acute awareness of the effect on the gut. You *feel* the spasms in your colon, and you will experience diarrhea if the spasms all go one way and constipation if the spasms go up and down the intestine, essentially trapping the stools in the bowel. It may feel as if you suddenly, urgently need to defecate, and it may be uncomfortable or even painful. These symptoms are *real* and are the direct result of your body's physical response to stress.

Many researchers have suggested that part of the problem in IBS is a disorder in the connection between the brain and the gut. That is, something goes wrong in the communication between the three different parts of the ANS (the enteric nervous system, the parasympathetic nervous system, and the sympathetic nervous system), and the gut reacts to environmental and psychological stressors much more violently than it should.

Not surprisingly, lots of research into IBS has shown that *stress* is very closely linked to IBS symptom severity. Again, this does *not* mean that your symptoms are "all in your head" or that you are just neurotic. Rather, we now understand a lot more about the *physical* effect psychological stress has on the digestive system, particularly in people with a predisposition to visceral hypersensitivity and abnormal intestinal motility.

GUT SYMPTOMS AS A STRESSOR

Of course, everyone has to deal with life stress. But when you throw gut symptoms into the mix, things that might be somewhat stressful (like a long family car trip or an important meeting) can become *hugely* stressful. That's because it's natural to worry about the possibility of having a flare-up. But here's the thing: just as the neurons in your intestinal wall may be sending more "problem signals" than they need to, you may be entertaining more "problem thoughts" than you need to.

People with gut problems often develop anxiety about the consequences of having GI symptoms. For example, many people worry about feeling embarrassed if they have to excuse themselves to go to the bathroom frequently. They worry about offending or disgusting people with smelly bowel movements or farts. They worry that they will be seen as unprofessional or incompetent if their gut acts up during the workday.

They worry that they will be viewed as weird or antisocial if they decline invitations to dinner or bring their own food to social events or public gatherings. They worry about annoying people and calling unwanted attention to themselves if they have to get up during a class, a movie, or a worship service. Beyond these social concerns, many people with gut problems truly fear getting stuck someplace without ready access to a bathroom. Trains, planes, cars, large malls, stadiums, theaters, or parks can all become anxiety provoking. A casual afternoon shopping with friends or catching a ball game begins to feel like a serious gamble.

"Can I make it through?"

"What if I have an attack?"

"What if I can't get to a bathroom quickly enough?"

Many people with gut problems become experts at scoping out potential bathroom locations. Some people even start consulting "bathroom finder" websites before they venture out of the house. Sometimes, just staying home seems like the safest course of action, but then you give up on life experiences that you would otherwise enjoy.

One of the things some people with IBS fear the most is losing control and having a bowel movement in their clothes. The actual incidence of *fecal incontinence* is hard to determine for several reasons. First, many people don't tell their doctor about it. Second, in the studies that have been done, the definition of fecal incontinence includes involuntary passing of *gas*. Yes, that's right, farting counts as "incontinence" in most studies. So even though some studies report prevalence rates of anywhere from 25 to 50 percent,* it's very difficult to interpret what those numbers actually

* Atarodi, S., Rafielian, S. & Whorwell, P.J. (2014). Faecal incontinence: The hidden scourge of irritable bowel syndrome. *BMJ Open Gastroenterology,* 1:e000002 doi:10.1136/bmjgast-2014-000002; and Longstreth, G.F. & Wolde-Tsadik, G. (1993). Irritable bowel-type symptoms in HMO examinees. Prevalence, demographics, and clinical correlates. *Digestive Diseases and Science, 38*(9), 1581–1589.

mean. Generally, *true* incontinence (that is, actually passing stool involuntarily) is quite rare, except in the very elderly and people with serious bowel diseases or a history of abdominal surgery or pelvic surgery in which the sphincter muscles were affected. Ironically, heavy laxative use in people with constipation-predominant IBS accounts for at least 10 percent of cases. Whatever the actual prevalence is, it's not hard to find "horror stories" on IBS websites told by people who really did experience this mishap at least once. In fact, it's not uncommon for IBS to *start* with a bout of food poisoning or a terrible stomach flu that led to extreme diarrhea and a single instance of fecal incontinence associated with illness. After the physical illness resolves, people are left with a terrible fear that their gut difficulties will continue. In people with visceral hypersensitivity, this can become a *self-fulfilling prophecy*. People notice every sensation, every twinge, every muscle spasm in their gut. These sensations make them anxious, as they anticipate the onset of more serious cramps or pain or urgent diarrhea. As soon as they get anxious, sympathetic and enteric nervous system activation starts, causing more roiling and cramping, and increasing the urge to defecate. Now they may start to worry about getting to a bathroom. They imagine having another episode of fecal incontinence, and this really gets the worry juices flowing. It would be humiliating! Horrible! Even *disastrous*! Before you know it, they dash out of the room, desperate to get to the bathroom "in time." In the majority of cases, people with IBS do *not* experience actual fecal incontinence. But they sure do worry about it a lot.

If you are actually experiencing incontinence currently, there are standard medical protocols to follow that may be able to diagnose the source of the problem, and there are interventions (including biofeedback training, pelvic floor exercises, surgery, and electrical stimulation) that can correct underlying problems. Ironically, one of the most common causes of fecal incontinence is *constipation*. This is counterintuitive, but it makes sense when you understand it. Hard, dry stools impact in the rectum, stretch the muscle walls, and weaken them. Loose, liquid stool then builds up behind the impacted hard stool and can "leak out" around the edges because the muscles are stretched and weak. This may actually be the result of long-term use of antidiarrheal medications like Pepto-Bismol®, Imodium, and Lomotil, which many people with diarrhea-predominant IBS use a lot. The long-term solution is to stop using those meds and dramatically increase soluble fiber in the diet (see Chapter 8, "Diet and IBS").

Most people with IBS who *fear* fecal incontinence have never actually experienced it. Yet they fear it a *lot*.

CHRONIC INFLAMMATION

A recent advance in our understanding of IBS is the role of chronic, low-grade inflammation and the degree to which stress and stress hormones contribute to the inflammatory process. *Inflammation* is the result of processes the body engages in to *protect* and heal itself from tissue damage or infection. In the short term, normal inflammation is quite helpful. Indeed, failure of the body to generate an inflammatory response is linked to some serious diseases and can make us more vulnerable to or can prolong infections. But *chronic inflammation* is clearly not good for us. In chronic inflammation, the inflammatory response is either too strong, goes on too long, or is directed at the wrong targets. Many diseases and conditions in modern society are actually the result of chronic inflammation that is misdirected in some way. Examples include allergies, asthma, rheumatoid arthritis, lupus, and multiple sclerosis, as well as the inflammatory bowel diseases like Crohn's and ulcerative colitis.

Recent research suggests that corticotrophin releasing factor (CRF), which is released by the brain when we are stressed, may modulate intestinal inflammation. There are CRF receptors in the brain *and* in the gut itself. CRF receptors may be components of the inflammatory processes in both IBD and post-infectious IBS. CRF is released in the brain in response to stressors and helps activate the hypothalamic-pituitary-adrenal (HPA) axis, a crucial part of the stress response system. Brain CRF also acts on the autonomic nervous system. In addition, the gut contains CRF sensors that contribute to stress-related exacerbation of both IBD and IBS. This shared vulnerability may be why IBD patients are more likely than the general population to develop IBS.

FRIENDLY BACTERIA AND THE HUMAN MICROBIOME

One final, and very intriguing, hypothesis about the cause of IBS and the IBDs is that they might be related to disruptions in the human microbiome—that is, the population of microorganisms that lives inside us. Throughout most of the history of modern medicine, bacteria have been seen as the enemy. Ever since Louis Pasteur conducted his famous experiments proving that germs caused many diseases, the "germ theory" of medicine has held sway. Germ theory turned out to be an incredibly powerful paradigm that shifted medicine away from mostly ineffective and often harmful interventions (like bloodletting) to the successful vanquishing of some of the most virulent and deadly diseases known to humanity, including smallpox, polio, and tuberculosis. The combination of vaccines that teach the immune system to fight viruses and bacteria, and antibiotics, which actually kill bacterial pathogens, has saved literally hundreds of millions of lives and spared many millions more the disfigurement and disability that used to be common hazards for all humans. Germ theory and modern industrial life, with indoor plumbing, clean running water, containment of sewage, and safety inspectors in food processing plants, have also dramatically reduced the impact of dangerous bacterial infections like cholera, salmonella, and E. coli. There is no doubt that germ theory, and the resulting war on germs, has benefited humankind enormously.

But there is a downside to all this antigerm fervor. There are very good reasons to believe that we have taken this one-sided view of germs too far, and we are actually now *hurting* ourselves with our endless efforts to disinfect and sterilize our environments. We are constantly advised to wash our hands, disinfect our cutting boards and kitchen counters, use hand sanitizers at every opportunity, and purchase innumerable products with antimicrobial chemicals embedded in them. This has had three unexpected and quite negative consequences. First, the excessive use of germicidal chemicals has spurred the evolution of *resistant super-bacteria*. Overprescription of antibiotics was routine medical practice for years. Only very recently have physicians, researchers, and medical organizations sounded the alarm about the rise of resistant strains of tuberculosis and other frightening bacteria like MRSA (methicillin-resistant Staphylococcus aureus). Indeed, the American Medical Association has recently issued a position statement warning *against* the use of antimicrobial agents like triclosan in consumer products such as hand sanitizer, dishwashing soap, and cutting boards. They cite evidence suggesting that such use is actually *harmful* to public health because it spurs the development of resistant bacteria.

But even more important for our purposes are the *other* unintended consequences of too much sterilization of our environment. First, those of us who live in the industrialized world are ending up with *dumb immune systems*. There is considerable evidence for the "hygiene hypothesis" that explains the dramatic rise in the incidence of a variety of autoimmune disorders in the developed world. It turns out that exposure to a wide range of microorganisms before age five is crucial to the development of the immune system. Parents of young children in day care may bemoan the many sniffles, coughs, and runny noses their kids come home with. But they should take heart in knowing that their kids are *much* less likely to develop asthma or serious allergies by the time they're fifteen than kids who stay home until they start kindergarten. When the immune system doesn't get to learn who the bad guys are and how to fight them, it grows up not being able to distinguish the bad guys from the good guys, or even the bad guys from the self. This has led to a dramatic rise in autoimmune disorders, including allergies, asthma, lupus, rheumatoid arthritis, and the inflammatory bowel diseases in the developed world. As one gastroenterologist I work with put it, "There's a thin line between dying of cholera and developing Crohn's." The incidence of inflammatory bowel diseases like Crohn's in developing countries in Asia, Africa, and South America is *tiny*.* Goat herders in Ethiopia *don't* get Crohn's disease, though they may well have intestinal worms. Amazingly, there are several small but promising clinical trials suggesting that a brief intestinal worm infestation may actually *cure* Crohn's disease—normalizing the immune system factors that cause the abnormal inflammatory process. Give the immune system a *real* threat to fight, and it stops attacking symbiotic bacteria and gut tissue. If we could just get past the "yuck" factor, it might become a common treatment for Crohn's.

The final unintended consequence of the war on germs is that we may well be killing off the very bacteria that we need to thrive. This is the most challenging part for most Westerners to accept, but we actually live symbiotically with trillions of bacteria *in our own bodies*. In fact, our bodies are composed of about ten microorganisms for every one human cell, and the vast majority of them live *in the gut*. Collectively known as *gut flora*, these microorganisms play a vital role in helping us digest our food, keeping pathogenic bacteria in check, educating the immune system, and *reducing* inflammation. Keeping these friendly bacterial populations healthy and in the right balance turns out to be crucial for overall and digestive health. Scientists have raised mice from birth in completely sterile environments. Their guts are pristine—no bacteria at all. And the mice are a mess. They're puny, weak, and can't digest food properly at

---

* Bernstein, C.N., Fried, M., Krabshuis, J.H., et al. Inflammatory bowel disease: A global perspective (2009, June). *World Gastroenterology Organisation Global Guidelines,* Downloaded from http://www.worldgastroenterology.org/guidelines/global-guidelines/inflammatory-bowel-disease-ibd/inflammatory-bowel-disease-ibd-english August 31, 2015

all. At least some cases of IBS may be the result of dramatic imbalances in the ecosystem of the gut flora. This helps explain why some people go on to develop post-infectious IBS, especially if they've been treated with vigorous regimens of broad-spectrum antibiotics.

For a while, there was hope that some IBS cases might be the result of *small intestine bacterial overgrowth (SIBO)* that contributed to gas, bloating, flatulence, intense discomfort, and alternating diarrhea and constipation. The solution, of course, according to germ theory, was an aggressive course of antibiotics. Unfortunately, that treatment does no better than placebo in the long run. Why? Because even if you kill some problematic bacteria, you're probably also killing *good* bacteria, and you've done nothing to reestablish the *balance* of the ecosystem in the gut. Imagine you have a white-tailed deer population that's out of control and wreaking havoc in a suburb. If you kill most of the deer, you've solved the problem only temporarily (and probably upset a lot of people in the community). Without natural predators (like wolves and cougars) and competitors (like elk and mule deer), the white-tailed deer will quickly repopulate, and you're right back where you started. The same thing happens in the microecosystem of the gut. Without good, helpful symbiotic bacteria to colonize the gut and work with us, killing off "bad" bacteria won't help. This may be why probiotics (which contain "live cultures" of symbiotic bacteria) have shown some promise in the management of IBS (see Chapter 8, "Diet and IBS").

The most dramatic example of the need for "good" bacteria in the gut comes from transplant surgery. When people with serious bowel problems required transplant surgery, physicians used to take great pains to wash and sterilize the donor intestinal tissue. This makes sense from a germ theory perspective. But it turned out to be a terrible idea. Believe it or not, allowing the donor tissue to retain its natural complement of symbiotic bacteria leads to *much* better outcomes for the recipient. A natural extension of this has been the development of a truly bizarre-*sounding* procedure called *fecal microbiota transplantation,* or FMT, in which stool from a healthy person is inserted via enema into the intestines of someone struggling with IBS, IBD, or a serious C. diff infection. After all, poop is actually about 30 percent bacteria. The outcome data on this procedure are growing and highly encouraging, especially in the case of C. diff infections. Long-term follow-up of these patients has shown a complete restoration of *normal gut flora* many months down the road, and the patients remain symptom free, often after a single treatment. Indeed, many mainstream gastroenterologists now suggest that FMT should be considered a front-line treatment for C. diff infections, and many more are recommending it for IBDs. The evidence for IBS is intriguing but less compelling, and we still need to conduct clinical trials before it becomes a mainstream treatment, but this approach is very promising and may offer long-term relief to people with serious GI problems in years to come.

In the meantime, however, there is still a great deal we can do to empower people to manage their GI problems more effectively and improve their quality of life dramatically.

SUMMARY

IBS seems to be caused by a combination of factors, some of which we tend to think of as biological (like intestinal motility, inflammation, and bacterial ecosystems), some of which are psychological (like emotional distress, worry, anxiety, and embarrassment), and some of which are environmental (like stressful life events). This is what IBS researchers refer to as the *biopsychosocial model* of IBS.

If you think about it, almost everything in our lives happens simultaneously *at all three levels*. Let's say you are supposed to go to your in-laws' house for dinner. You are getting ready to go, and you're thinking about the last time you were there—how your mother-in-law was critical of you and how she and your father-in-law sometimes snipe at each other. You're feeling a little tense. Then you notice a small, crampy twinge in your gut. Could this be a flare-up? Maybe you shouldn't have had that salad at lunch. Maybe you should try to go to the bathroom before you get in the car. But what if it takes a while? Then you'll be late, and your spouse will be frustrated and annoyed. Maybe you should just suck it up and go. But then what if you *really* have to go halfway there? Is there a gas station along the way with a restroom that's not too disgusting? Or what if you have to run to the bathroom the instant you arrive? What if you stink up their powder room? You can always say you're sick. But that will just give your mother-in-law something else about you to criticize. By now your gut is cramping in earnest. It hurts, and you know there's no way you can get in the car without going to the bathroom first.

What's going on here? Clearly, there's an *environmental* or *social stressor* at work. Obviously, your in-laws are a bit difficult to deal with. Anticipating dealing with this stressor is causing you apprehension and anxiety—that's the *psychological distress* part of the equation. But psychological distress translates directly into sympathetic nervous system arousal, which leads to an inflammatory stress response, which interacts with the enteric nervous system to cause some sensory overload and abnormal motility in a gut that's prone to inflammation and may not have enough helpful bacteria onboard—that's the *biological* piece. This feeds back through *visceral hypersensitivity* to ensure that you notice the twinges and spasms. But the twinges and spasms now become stressors in and of themselves, triggering a new onslaught of worrisome thoughts, which, in turn, trigger more arousal and inflammation, which then increase the physical discomfort and the urgent need to defecate. Before you know it, you're having a full-fledged IBS attack and you feel horribly sick. Your spouse is alternately sympathetic and annoyed. You and your spouse may cancel the dinner, leading to bad feelings all around. Or you may go, feeling drained and exhausted, and then only pick at dinner, fearful of bringing on another attack and further alienating your difficult mother-in-law.

The point is that the constellation of symptoms we call irritable bowel syndrome is really the end result of *all these processes* put together and happening at the same time. It's sort of like a perfect storm of stressors, worry, experience, and fears interacting with a vulnerable GI system.

The good news is that there are ways to intervene quite effectively to reduce the impact of gut symptoms on your life and to give you considerable relief from this constant GI distress. This entire program is designed to empower you—to teach you skills to manage stress effectively, to reduce the impact of stress on your gut, and to reduce the degree to which your life is limited and defined by having to manage your gut symptoms. So let's get started!

SUGGESTED ACTIVITIES

1. Complete the self-report questionnaires in Appendices D and E. This will give you a sense of how much you suffer from *visceral hypersensitivity* and the degree to which your beliefs about your gut symptoms themselves have become real stressors for you.

2. Keep a daily symptom log this week to assess the severity of your symptoms on a day-to-day basis, and to collect information about whether particular stressors are associated with gut symptoms for you. A sample symptom log can be found in Appendix F.

Chapter Three

RELAXATION TRAINING

It's important to remember that stress makes GI symptoms worse for very straightforward biological reasons. All three parts of the autonomic nervous system (sympathetic, parasympathetic, and enteric) talk to each other and work in concert with each other. If you are stressed, the parasympathetic system gets quiet, the sympathetic system goes into overdrive, and the enteric system reacts to the signals the sympathetic system is sending it (through chemicals like corticotropin releasing factor, or CRF). So stress has a direct, *physical* impact on your body and your gut.

The good news is that you can actually learn to turn on the *parasympathetic* nervous system consciously and intentionally. The parasympathetic nervous system is the one that allows for *resting and digesting* in peace. It's the opposite of sympathetic activation (*fight or flight or freeze*), which is the body's response to stress. So turning on the parasympathetic nervous system is equivalent to turning *off* the sympathetic nervous system. The behavioral exercises that follow are designed to reduce the physical impact of stress on your body and your GI system. When practiced regularly and used effectively, they can actually reduce the severity of GI symptoms. But keep in mind that this program is not like a pill or medicine you take in the short term. This is a training program designed to teach you a set of skills you can use for the rest of your life to manage stress effectively. If you don't practice these, they definitely won't do you any good.

There are three basic types of relaxation exercises:

1. Deep Breathing
2. Progressive Muscle Relaxation
3. Relaxing Imagery

Many people find that they gravitate to one or two of them but don't much care for the other(s). It's important to try all three types at least a few times to see if you can get the feel for them and see if they work for you. My own personal favorite is deep breathing. Done correctly, deep breathing can really take the edge off sympathetic arousal. It can also be done discreetly, anytime and anywhere—in the car, in a meeting, after lunch, you name it. When you get good at it, just two to three deep breaths—about thirty seconds' total time investment—can lower your heart rate and blood pressure, suppress adrenaline and cortisol (a major stress hormone), and relax the smooth muscles in your colon.

Some people swear by progressive muscle relaxation. They like the structure of thinking about each major muscle group in turn, alternately tensing and relaxing each muscle. They find that the immediate feeling of warmth and release in the muscles is very relaxing and reassuring. It's a very concrete exercise, and it makes you feel that you're really *doing* something to help your body relax.

Other people, especially those high in imaginal ability, love using relaxing imagery to "take them away" from their stress. Imaginal ability is the degree to which you can create mental images that feel real and vivid to you. The more real your imagery feels, the easier it is to get "caught up" in it and the more relaxing it will be. Imagery can work especially well for people with IBS who feel that their body has become the "enemy." If you don't trust your body anymore and feel as if it betrays you and causes you nothing but pain and aggravation, deep breathing and progressive muscle relaxation may be frustrating and counterproductive because they focus you on and in your body. If this is true for you, by all means use imagery instead for a month or two. But as this program starts to work, it might be worth coming back to deep breathing and trying it again.

No matter which type of relaxation exercise ends up being the most useful to you, give them all a try.

1. DEEP BREATHING

Ever heard the advice to "just take a deep breath"? It sounds like good advice, but unfortunately it doesn't work very well for most people. That's because there are two very different ways of breathing. One of them—chest breathing (where your shoulders go up and your upper chest expands)—isn't really deep breathing at all, but it's what most people do when you ask them to take a deep breath. It's what most people do at the doctor's office when their physician says, "Now take a deep breath." Try it—notice what you actually do when you try to "take a deep breath." Does your chest rise? Do your shoulders move up toward your ears? Taking that kind of breath will *not* help you relax. In fact, believe it or not, it will probably make you *more* tense. That's because chest breathing tends to *activate* the sympathetic nervous system, and that's not what we want!

Instead, try this. Stand up. Put your hand on your stomach with your belly button in the curve between your thumb and pointer finger. Now just contract your tummy muscles so your hand moves inward. You're not pressing in with your hand, but if your hand is resting lightly in the right place, it should move in and out as you contract that muscle. Don't worry about breathing yet. Just find that muscle, and keep contracting it over and over until you feel some muscle "burn" just under your rib cage (about six or seven times should do it). Feel it?

Now try to use that muscle to squeeze the air out of your lungs. As you contract the muscle, exhale sharply, as if you were blowing out a candle. Do this two or three times, then take a break for a few breaths, and try it again until you get the hang of it. (If you start to get dizzy, just stop and breathe normally for about fifteen seconds.)

Now do the same thing—use the muscle to squeeze the air out of your lungs, but instead of exhaling sharply, exhale *slowly* over a count of 4. After you finish exhaling, just relax, and *let yourself inhale*. Try to do this four or five times in a row, very slowly. You should be able to count to 4 while you exhale, count to 4 again while you relax (and inhale), then hold your breath for a few counts (as many as 4 would be great) before exhaling again. There's a rhythm to this:

> exhale—2—3—4, relax—2—3—4,
> hold your breath—2—3—4,
>
> exhale—2—3—4, relax—2—3—4,
> hold your breath—2—3—4,
>
> exhale—2—3—4, and so on.

Got it? You should find that as you relax after exhaling, you just inhale deeply and slowly without having to think about it too much. Now try again, and this time put one hand on your chest, and the other on your belly. You should find that the hand on your belly moves in and out with each exhale/inhale, while the hand on your chest doesn't move much at all. This is called *diaphragmatic,* or deep belly, breathing. Done correctly, diaphragmatic breathing actually *turns on* the parasympathetic nervous system and *turns off* the sympathetic nervous system. If you're doing it deeply and slowly, you should be taking between four and five breaths per minute, and you should feel warm and relaxed, and not dizzy at all. If you start to feel dizzy, you're probably breathing too fast. Just hold your breath a little longer after each inhale.

It may feel very awkward and unnatural at first, but I guarantee your body knows how to do it. It's what you naturally do when you're asleep. (Remember *rest and digest?* Sleeping is all about parasympathetic nervous system control.) The trick is to learn how to harness this consciously so that you can control it and get the good effects anytime you need a little help managing stress. If you're having trouble getting the feel for it, try practicing lying down. This makes it easier for some people.

Being able to consciously control your body's stress response is incredibly empowering for most people. So it's definitely worth practicing this until you get the hang of it. When you get good at it, you should be able to lower your blood pressure and heart rate, at least a little bit, at will. I always have fun when I go to the doctor. I practice deep breathing while I'm waiting for the assistant to come in and take my blood pressure. They're always surprised when it is 100/70. Occasionally (if I have to wait a while) I can get it down to 90/50. That *really* wigs them out! I've been practicing this for years now, but it should take only a few weeks for you to be able to lower your own heart rate and even your blood pressure with just four to five deep breaths. This very obvious evidence that you're reducing the body's stress response can be very encouraging. So give it a try!

2. PROGRESSIVE MUSCLE RELAXATION

Progressive muscle relaxation involves systematically tensing and relaxing the major muscle groups of the body. It may sound a little crazy to *tense* your muscles if you're trying to relax, but we're counting on the fact that tensing your muscles for about ten seconds actually leads to muscle *fatigue*. When you stop tensing the muscle, not only will it relax, it will actually get *more* relaxed than it normally is because the muscle fibers are tired. This should leave the muscle feeling quite lax, but also warm and vital.

Try to tense each major muscle group, in order, for about ten seconds each. Pay attention to how the muscles feel when they are tensed, compared to how they feel when you release the tension and let them relax. You should wait at least ten to fifteen seconds between working on each muscle group.

In general, start with a muscle group on one side of your body, then work on the same muscle group on the other side of the body.

1. Sitting in a comfortable chair, hold your right arm out over your lap, make a fist, bend it up toward the ceiling, and tense the lower right arm and wrist muscles as tightly as you can for ten seconds. Then relax your arm and let it drop into your lap. Now do the same thing with your left arm.

2. Bring your right hand up to your shoulder and tense the muscles in your upper arm, as if you were a bodybuilder showing off your biceps. Tense and hold tightly for ten seconds, then release. Now do the same thing with your left arm.

3. Hold your right leg out in front of you, point your toes, and tense your calf muscle as tightly as you can. Hold for ten seconds and then release. Then do the same thing with your left leg.

4. Extend your right leg straight out, flex your foot (point your toes toward the ceiling) and tense your thigh muscle as tightly as you can for ten seconds, then release. Do the same thing with your left leg.

5. Now put your knees together, squeeze your thighs together, and clench the muscles in your bottom as tightly as you can for ten seconds. Then release.

6. Still sitting in your chair, round your back by pulling your abdominal muscles in as tightly as you can and press the small of your back into the back of the chair. Hold for ten seconds and then release.

7. Stand up, clasp your hands together behind your back, and pull your hands down and out behind you, pulling your shoulder blades together as far

as you can. This should tighten the muscles in your back while simultaneously stretching the muscles in your chest. Hold for ten seconds and release.

8. Now hold your right arm in front of you across your chest so that your right hand juts out past your left shoulder. Grab your right elbow with your left hand, and pull your arm into your chest. Hold for ten seconds and release. Now do the same thing with your left arm, grabbing your left elbow with your right hand.

9. Drop your head down in front and pull your shoulders forward and down. Hold for ten seconds and release.

10. Finally, tense the muscles in your forehead and face by lifting your eyebrows up toward your hairline and opening your eyes as widely as you can. Hold for ten seconds and release.

A nice way to combine imagery and muscle relaxation is to use imagery to help you visualize a warm, relaxing feeling slowly moving up your body from your toes to the very top of your head. Instead of systematically tensing and relaxing your major muscles, you just focus on very small body parts in sequence, feeling them and trying to imagine letting all the tension go from that particular body part. Some people like to visualize a warm, golden light warming each part, in turn, until your whole body is bathed in relaxing warmth and you feel entirely limp and heavy, like honey in the sun. One of the tricks to this exercise is to try to relax body parts you don't normally think you can control (like your big toe or your hips or your ears). This helps you avoid the pitfall of inadvertently tensing a muscle just because you're focusing on it.

Start with the big toe on your right foot. Then move to the big toe on your left foot. Slowly change your focus to the rest of the toes, followed by the ball of your foot, the arch of your foot, the heel, and the ankle, going back and forth between left and right. Really take a second or two to focus your attention on that particular part of your body. When's the last time you focused on the feelings in your left heel? Let your mind center in that part for a moment, feeling the tension draining out, before you move on to the next body part. Move up your leg, imagining first the shin and then the calf of each leg being bathed in warm, golden light. Imagine your knees relaxing in front and in back. Take your time. Then imagine your thighs relaxing, then your hips, your bottom, and the small of your back. Move up your back to your shoulder blades, and up through your shoulders and down your arms to your elbows, your forearms, your wrist, your thumbs, and each finger in turn. Then come back up to your neck, and imagine the warm light relaxing first your chin, then your lips, your nose, your ears, your eyebrows, and your hair. By the time you've made it up to the top of your head, you should feel warm and limp and very languid. Ideally, you'll be doing slow diaphragmatic breathing, too, without even having realized that you're doing it!

3. RELAXING IMAGERY

Another thing a lot of people find relaxing is to imagine themselves in a place that they find very soothing and peaceful. For some people, the beach is perfect. Other people like to imagine themselves in the woods, or on top of a mountain, or in their grandmother's kitchen, or in a luxurious hotel suite with a private hot tub, or even floating around in a warm, lavender cloud. Whatever image you choose, make sure it feels like a safe, peaceful place to *you*. You should also pick something that you can imagine vividly and in detail, using the four senses of sight, hearing, touch, and smell. For example, if you're imagining being at the beach, try to see the play of light and shadow on the sand and notice how the color and shapes in the sand change as you walk down toward the water. The sand starts out dry, soft, and warm, with big, shapeless dimples where people have walked. As you approach the water, the sand gets darker, cooler, flatter, and slightly harder. When you get all the way down to the water, the sand gets squishy and wet. Listen to the waves crashing or lapping at the sand, and the sound of seabirds calling, and the rustling of the wind in the dune grasses. Smell the clean, tangy, salty smell of the sea. Feel the warm sun on your back, the cool breeze on your cheek, the soft sand underfoot, or the water slipping around your toes. Involve yourself in the image. Imagine running along the beach, or scooping up handfuls of water and watching the sunlight shatter into a million diamonds as you throw the water up into the air. The more involved, detailed, and vivid you can make the image, the more relaxing the exercise will be.

A nice way to combine this imagery with deep breathing is to imagine the waves rolling in to the beach in time with your breath. Watch each wave as it begins to surge, comes up in a crest, crashes onto the beach, and then gets pulled back out to sea, sucking at the pebbles and licking at the sand. You can imagine inhaling as the wave surges and crests, exhaling as it crashes and flows back out, and then pause for a count or two as the next wave begins to surge.

SUMMARY

In Chapter 2, "What's Causing My Gut Symptoms?," we mapped out the biological reasons that stress exacerbates physical symptoms and discomfort in the gut. Because of the powerful neurological connections between the brain and the gut, stress management is an important part of the treatment of IBS. One key part of stress management is behavioral—relaxation exercises that actually reduce the biological impact of chronic stress on our bodies. There are three basic types of relaxation exercises you can learn.

1. Deep Breathing
2. Progressive Muscle Relaxation
3. Relaxing Imagery

Most people find that they gravitate most naturally to one or another. Some people love deep breathing. They find it easy to learn, they can do it unobtrusively, and it quickly reduces stress and the physical arousal and discomfort associated with stress. On the other hand, trying to focus on breathing is boring or confusing for some people. They just can't seem to get the hang of it, at least not when they're trying to do it consciously. Some people love muscle relaxation. Other people find that it just focuses their attention on all their aches and pains and even heightens visceral sensitivity. If you feel like your body has become your enemy and betrays you at every turn, then focus on imagery, at least at the beginning. Most people find that they prefer one over the other two, or that a combination of two works well, but they hate the third one. The point is that you need to experiment until you find what works well for *you*.

Relaxation is a learned skill, like learning to ride a bicycle. With regular practice you become better at it. If you cannot, or will not, practice regularly, then you probably won't get much benefit from it. Once you learn this skill, however (and it usually takes just a few weeks to get good at it), it's something you'll be able to use to help you manage and reduce the physical impact of stress for the rest of your life. Even a thirty-second time-out during a stressful day to take two or three deep breaths and imagine yourself on the beach (or whichever peaceful place works for you) can do wonders for reducing your body's response to stress.

SUGGESTED ACTIVITIES

1. Practice deep breathing, progressive muscle relaxation, and relaxing imagery at least once a day, every day for a week, for ten to fifteen minutes. Lots of people like to do it shortly before bedtime, since it's very soothing and often helps them fall asleep. In fact, some people initially find it easier to practice deep breathing when they're lying down.

2. In addition to practicing the techniques, keep some notes about how it's going. Over the week, take a few moments to write a bit in the box on page 52 about how the relaxation exercises are going for you. Taking the time to write about your experiences can help you think about what you've learned and can point you in the right direction as you continue developing these skills.

MY EXPERIENCES WITH RELAXATION EXERCISES

You should continue practicing relaxation exercises at least three to four days a week for the rest of the program. Feel free to use only the components that work well for you.

Chapter Four

THE COGNITIVE MODEL OF STRESS MANAGEMENT

Behavioral management of stress (through things like relaxation exercises) is great, but it will get you only so far. Relaxation can reduce only the physical impact of stress you're already experiencing. Wouldn't it be better to reduce the actual stress itself?

You may have already tried to do this by curtailing certain activities (like traveling, shopping, or going to shows) or avoiding certain situations (like restaurants, parties, or other social gatherings, especially if they involve food). The problem with this strategy is that you end up missing out on *life*. Really living means being involved in life, not avoiding it. So rather than reducing stress by trying to *avoid* stressful situations, I'd like to teach you a better way to reduce stress by making potentially distressing situations less stressful to begin with.

Try the following exercise:

Imagine that you are walking down the street, and you see a casual friend walking on the other side of the street going in the opposite direction. You wave. Your friend does not wave back. Try your best to visualize such a scene as vividly as possible.

How do you feel? Take a moment to think about this, and try to identify what would go through your mind and what kind of emotions you might experience if you found yourself in this situation. Write down your reactions in the box below.

HOW WOULD I REACT IF I FOUND MYSELF IN THIS SITUATION?

Interestingly, different people might have lots of different reactions to this situation. Some people might be angry. Others might be sad. Still others might feel anxious. Some might feel faintly amused. Others might feel nothing at all. How can different people respond so incredibly differently to what appears to be the exact same situation?

The key, of course, is that it depends on what the person is *thinking* about the situation. If you think to yourself, "Look at that arrogant, snooty so-and-so. I can't believe she would just ignore me that way!," you are likely to feel angry. If, on the other hand, you think to yourself, "Wow—she must really not like me. Something must be wrong with me. I'm uninteresting, unattractive, geeky—I suck . . . ," you are likely to feel sad or even depressed. If you think to yourself, "Ohmygosh! I must have really screwed up to make her angry with me. I wonder what I did wrong? How am I going to face her this weekend?," you are likely to feel anxious. On the other hand, if you think to yourself, "I guess she didn't see me. Oh well. I'll say hi to her next time I see her," then you're not likely to feel much of anything. But if you add the thought, "Gosh, I wonder if other people saw me waving at nobody and think I'm crazy?," then you might feel embarrassed.

The point is that it is not really the objective situation *itself* that determines how we feel. All the people above experienced exactly the same objective reality. They waved, and their friend did not wave back. Their emotional response was determined by their *beliefs* about the situation. These thoughts, also known as *cognitions*, are very powerful. They cause us to feel emotions and even act in certain ways based on our beliefs about events. If you think the person is being deliberately mean and ignoring you, you may feel angry, and you may act coldly toward the person the next time you see her. If you think that there is something wrong with you, or that you screwed up somehow, you may feel sad or anxious, and you may cry or try to avoid the person. The key thing to understand is the connection between the objective situation, your beliefs, and your feelings.

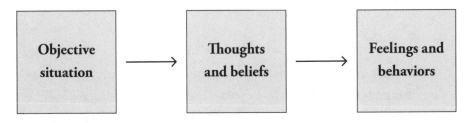

Now try to apply this to a real situation from your own life.

Think about a recent situation or event that was stressful for you—something recent enough that you can remember it reasonably well. This may or may not also be a situation in which your gut acted up. Try to describe the situation as objectively as possible in the box below.

> **DESCRIBE A RECENT SITUATION THAT YOU EXPERIENCED AS STRESSFUL.**

Now try to identify what you *thought* in response to the situation. Examples include any *beliefs* you had about the situation—like about why it happened or how it was likely to end, any *judgments* you made about yourself or others (e.g., "I really screwed up" or "I should or shouldn't have . . ." or "What a jerk he was") or any *predictions* you might have made (e.g., "I bet I failed the exam" or "She must think I'm really stupid"), and so on. Write down these thoughts in the box below.

WHAT THOUGHTS DID YOU HAVE IN RESPONSE TO THE SITUATION?

Now try to identify all the different emotions you felt. Be careful here! In English, it's perfectly grammatically correct to say, "I feel like I failed the exam" but that's a thought—not a feeling. You are *thinking* that you might have failed the exam—so that belongs in the thoughts box, not the emotions box. That thought may make you *feel* sad and anxious. Sadness and anxiety are *emotions* and they go in the feelings box. Some people have a lot of difficulty identifying their emotions. Here's a cheat sheet of emotion words to help you out. (We're focusing on negative or unpleasant emotions here, since we're mostly concerned about stressful experiences. There are lots of positive emotions, too, of course.)

NEGATIVE EMOTION CHEAT SHEET

SADNESS	FEAR	ANGER
Unhappy	Apprehensive	Annoyed
Upset	Worried	Frustrated
Sad	Anxious	Irritated
Discouraged	Nervous	Aggravated
Miserable	Scared	Angry
Depressed	Terrified	Furious
Hopeless	Petrified	Enraged

Now, thinking about the situation you identified and the thoughts you had, fill in the feelings you experienced in the box on the next page. You can certainly use words that aren't on the cheat sheet if they seem to capture your feelings more accurately; just be sure you're describing emotions, not thoughts. If the situation also seemed to lead to an increase in your gut symptoms, note that in this box, too.

WHAT FEELINGS DID YOU HAVE IN RESPONSE TO THE SITUATION?

Ideally, you should be able to see the connection between your thoughts and your feelings. In fact, every feeling in the feelings box should be tied to at least one thought in the thoughts box. If there are feelings you identified that don't seem to be tied to a thought, it probably means you haven't really identified all the thoughts you had. For example, imagine that you have just taken an important exam or test of some kind. You might do the following analysis of what happened.

SITUATION	THOUGHTS	FEELINGS
I took the exam.	I think I did badly.	Anxious Disappointed Hopeless Guilty

If you try to connect each of the feelings to a thought, here's what happens.

SITUATION	THOUGHTS	FEELINGS
I took the exam.	I think I did badly. ⟶	Anxious ↘ Disappointed Hopeless Guilty

It may be obvious why you feel anxious and disappointed. But why do you feel hopeless and guilty? To understand where those feelings are coming from, you have to dig a little deeper into what you were thinking.

SITUATION	THOUGHTS	FEELINGS
I took the exam.	I think I did badly. ⟶ This means I won't get what I want professionally. ⟶ I screwed up by not preparing more. ⟶	Anxious Disappointed Hopeless Guilty

When the analysis is complete, you should be able to draw an arrow from a thought to a feeling for every feeling you experienced. Try this now with the situation from your own life that you wrote about above. Be sure that each of the feelings you experienced is "explained" by a thought.

SITUATION	THOUGHTS	FEELINGS

The interesting thing about feelings is that they are not right or wrong. They just *are*. That is, they are the inevitable consequences of our beliefs and thoughts. Beliefs, however, *can* be right or wrong. We call these worksheets "thought records," rather than situation or feeling records, because we want to emphasize that identifying and questioning your thoughts is the key to reducing unnecessary stress in your life.

> Just because we believe something doesn't make it true,
> even if we believe it very strongly and feel very certain that
> we are right.

Think back to the hypothetical situation I presented at the beginning of the chapter. A person might be thinking all kinds of negative, upsetting things about why her friend didn't wave back to her. She may be absolutely convinced that the friend ignored her on purpose, and she may be very upset as a result. If in fact the friend just didn't see her, then she will be upset *for no reason*. That is, she will be experiencing a whole lot of unnecessary stress. There is an objective reality out there. Either her friend saw her or she didn't.

How can you tell? In the heat of the moment, it can sometimes be hard or even impossible to know. That's why we usually just accept our first gut response, or *automatic thought*, without closely examining or questioning it.

The key to reducing unnecessary stress in your life is to make sure that your beliefs are as accurate as possible. All of us jump to conclusions sometimes. If you can catch yourself, and try to see situations in alternative ways, you may save yourself a lot of pain. The problem is, we usually don't think about *benign alternatives*, or other ways of looking at the situation that are less upsetting, once we've started to have an emotional reaction. If you're already angry and sad because you think you're being ignored, it may not occur to you that maybe your friend didn't see you. The instant you have a negative thought, it may set off a cascade of reactions, including both negative emotions and physical symptoms. This makes it hard to think objectively and clearly in the heat of the moment. One way to practice this is to think about the situation later and see if other, less stressful ways of thinking about it occur to you. For example, our hypothetical person might have done the following analysis:

SITUATION	THOUGHTS	FEELINGS	BENIGN ALTERNATIVE
My friend did not wave to me on the street.	She's ignoring me. She must not like me that much. Maybe she doesn't think I'm cool enough to be friends with. People are so judgmental and cruel.	Embarrassed Sad Frustrated Angry	Maybe she just didn't see me.

Now try to do a similar analysis with the situation you described from your own life. See if you can come up with *benign alternatives* to the *automatic thoughts* you identified. Try to list at least one benign alternative in the box below.

SITUATION	THOUGHTS	FEELINGS	BENIGN ALTERNATIVE

People run into several different problems when they start learning to do this. Occasionally, they just can't think of any other way to interpret or understand the situation than their initial take on it. There are a couple of ways to solve this. First, imagine that a friend came to you with a similar situation. What would you say to him? Often it is easier to see alternatives for other people than for ourselves. Another way to deal with this is to run it by an actual friend or partner, and see if she has another take on it. Try not to bias her by telling her right off the bat what *you* thought. Just describe the situation as objectively as possible, and ask her what she thinks might have been going on. Even if she doesn't come up with a *benign* alternative, she may come up with a *different* set of thoughts than you had. The very fact that there is at least one other way of looking at the situation may help you come up with more.

One alternative that often doesn't work very well is to just say the opposite of the original thought. For example, if your boss was short with you in the hallway and didn't smile, you might be thinking that he or she is angry with you or dissatisfied with your work. That thought is pretty anxiety provoking, and will probably stress you out. It's not very powerful to just say, "Well, maybe he's not angry with me." This is just contradicting the worrisome thought. It's not really providing an *alternative explanation* for your boss's behavior, so it's not very reassuring. It would be much more powerful to remind yourself, "Oh right, she's got a big presentation to make to the VP tomorrow—maybe she's just stressed about that." Or, if you don't *know* of anything that might explain it, try to remind yourself that there may be many other alternatives, like "Maybe there's something going on in his personal life or maybe he just got reamed by someone else. It could have nothing to do with me." Most of us have been short with someone at some point because we were stressed out about something that had nothing to do with him or her. This is more believable than the simple "Maybe she's not angry at me" because it doesn't ignore the actual objective behavior—your boss did not smile or engage you in conversation. It takes the objective behavior into account, but then provides a more benign *explanation* of why it happened and what it meant.

Another problem that people run into is that they can think of benign alternatives, but they just don't *believe* them. "Sure, I suppose it's possible that she just didn't see me, but I don't really think so." Something about the situation convinces you that the more stressful interpretation is the correct one. You may be right. How can you tell? *Examine the evidence.* In the waving friend situation, you might think back to the last contact you had with that friend. If she called you two days ago to set up a get-together over the weekend, it's unlikely that she's deliberately ignoring you. If, on the other hand, you've left two voice mails and a text message that haven't been answered, she may be trying to tell you something. Sometimes we have screwed up. Sometimes other people have. It may be that it's appropriate to feel distressed about the situation. The question then becomes what to do to fix the problem. Here, again, you will find that you have thoughts and beliefs that make you feel more or less optimistic and inclined to take action. Thoughts like "It won't work" or "She'll never listen" or "It's hopeless" or "I can't do it" are likely to undermine your efforts to resolve a problem. The basic lesson here is that, once again, your beliefs are what matter most in shaping your emotional response and your behavior.

One final type of difficulty people sometimes have with this sort of exercise is that they can think of an alternative—it makes sense; they may even believe it intellectually—but at the "gut level" they still feel awful. You still feel distressed about the situation and can't shake it. This is usually a clue that there are some other thoughts you haven't identified yet. For example, you might believe that that particular friend didn't see you on that particular occasion. But what you're really thinking about is how few friends you have, how isolated you feel, and how lonely you'll be this weekend—again. If that's the underlying thought, then convincing yourself that *that friend* didn't see you from across the street won't make you feel any better, because your encounter with that friend is not *really* why you're feeling so anxious and depressed.

Sometimes when people first hear about these techniques, they think it's a question of learning how to see the glass as "half-full" instead of seeing it as "half-empty." But cognitive interventions are asking you to do something entirely different. In cognitive therapy, we are asking you to look at the glass and say to yourself:

"It's a twelve-ounce glass with six ounces of water in it."

This response is completely, objectively *true*. Both of the traditional responses to this problem are *biased*. One is biased negatively (the glass is half-empty) and the other is biased positively (the glass is half-full). But the most objective way of looking at it involves no bias at all. How you *feel* about the glass with six ounces of water in it should depend on how thirsty you are! If all you need to do is swallow a vitamin, six ounces of water is more than enough and it's all good. If you just finished an intense workout and are very thirsty, six ounces of water won't be nearly enough. Now you have a concrete problem to solve—you need to get some more water.

That is to say, cognitive interventions are not about "pretending" that things are going well if they're not. In fact, this wouldn't help even if you tried it, because you wouldn't believe it. Rather, cognitive interventions are about helping you learn to see the world as *accurately* and *objectively* as possible. The problem is that many, many people *do* have negative biases or filters that they use to interpret situations in their lives. If you do this routinely and without realizing it, you will be a lot more stressed than you need to be. If you have been entertaining lots of negatively biased automatic thoughts, then seeing the world more accurately should bring about a great deal of relief. In other words:

Don't believe everything you think.

Another nice metaphor for understanding this approach is the following. Imagine that there is a bright yellow lemon sitting on the table in front of you. Now imagine that you have put on a pair of sunglasses with deep-blue lenses. What color is the lemon? If you think back to your basic art classes in elementary school, you'll remember that yellow + blue = green, and you'll say that that the lemon is green. But here's the thing. *Is* the lemon green? Just because the lemon *looks* green to you doesn't mean it has turned green in the real world. The lemon is, of course, still yellow. If you slice into it and taste it, it will still be a sour lemon, not a bitter green lime. Now imagine that you take off the dark-blue glasses and put on lovely rosy-red-colored glasses. Of course, red + yellow = orange. But by now, you know that just because the lemon *looks* orange to you doesn't mean it *is* orange. It's still yellow. If you slice into it now, it will still be a sour lemon, not a nice sweet orange. Negatively biased thinking is like those dark-blue sunglasses. It makes things *appear* worse than they actually are. On the other hand, falsely optimistic thinking is like rose-colored glasses. It makes things appear better than they actually are. I don't want you to do either one. I want you to see the world the way it actually *is*.

Occasionally, people have a very difficult time even understanding why an event or a future possibility has upset them so much. They may be able to identify perfectly sensible, benign, alternative ways to think about it, but the deep, gut-level distress doesn't seem to go away. Again, this is a clue that they haven't really identified the truly distressing thought. If this happens to you, then an interesting question to ask yourself is "What's the worst part about this?" or "What would be so terrible about that?" Oftentimes, there's some other, deeper belief that is distressing you. For example, you may believe in your heart of hearts that it is totally unacceptable to screw up. If you're the guilty party, it may say something terrible about you. If the other person is the guilty party, it may signal betrayal and probably means the permanent end of a friendship. This deeper belief—"it is totally unacceptable to screw up"—should now become the target of your analysis. Is there a benign alternative? There had better be, since human beings are not perfect, and screwing up occasionally is inevitable!

Although some people do encounter these difficulties with this kind of exercise, sometimes just putting the thought down in black and white is enough to help you gain a bit more objectivity. A common experience of people doing this sort of exercise for the first time is that the minute they say an automatic thought out loud, or write it down, it starts to look exaggerated and even silly. You can recognize immediately that the thought doesn't really make sense. It just doesn't bear up under scrutiny, so you reject it and start to feel better. That's the beauty of this. Since those thoughts usually go totally unexamined and unquestioned, the simple act of questioning them is sometimes enough to make us feel significantly better.

One final thing to note: It's very common for people to notice themes in their thoughts and feelings. For example, you might notice that you often respond to very different situations with the same basic feeling—maybe anger or anxiety. You may also find that you tend to have very similar thoughts across a range of situations. For example, take three different stressors that lots of people might experience—a bad haircut; a mediocre performance review at work; and a partner, family member, or roommate leaving dirty dishes in the sink. Here are two different sample thought records from two different people.

Amanda

SITUATIONS	THOUGHTS	FEELINGS	BENIGN ALTERNATIVE
Bad haircut	I look like an idiot. I can't believe how ugly I feel. I'm so unattractive. I never look good, no matter how much money I spend.	Sad Worth-less Anxious	Maybe I didn't explain what I wanted very well. I just expected my stylist to figure it out. Next time, I'll explain what I want more clearly. If I get another bad cut, I'll just find another hairdresser.
Mediocre perfor-mance review at work	I'm just incom-petent. My boss thinks I'm an idiot. I never seem to do well, no matter how hard I try.	Sad Worth-less Anxious	We're all really overworked right now because of all the lay-offs. I'm trying to do the work of two and a half people here! No wonder I can't get it all done. Maybe my boss and I need to sit down and have a meeting about reason-able expectations.
Dirty dishes	I'm such a sucker. Why do I always end up doing the dishes? I must have *doormat* written on my forehead.	Sad Worth-less Anxious	Maybe I haven't really communicated clearly about how important this is to me.

Roger

SITUATIONS	THOUGHTS	FEELINGS	BENIGN ALTERNATIVE
Bad haircut	God, that barber is an idiot. I can't believe what a bad job he did. Was he paying any attention at all? I shouldn't even have paid him.	Angry Frustrated	Maybe I didn't explain what I wanted very well. I just expected him to remember from last time. Next time, I'll explain what I want more clearly.
Mediocre performance review at work	My boss is an idiot. I'm working overtime on stuff I wasn't even hired to do, she's too lazy to get me the reports in time to do a good job, and she has the gall to give *me* a bad review!	Angry Frustrated	We're *all* really overworked and stressed right now because of all the layoffs, including my boss. Maybe she and I need to sit down and have a meeting about reasonable expectations.
Dirty dishes	Argh! I can't believe they left the dirty dishes again. That is so incredibly inconsiderate and lazy.	Angry Frustrated	Maybe I haven't really communicated clearly about how important this is to me.

You'll notice that Amanda tends to blame herself when things go wrong. She sees herself as "an idiot" or "incompetent" or "a sucker." As a result, Amanda often feels sad, worthless, and a bit anxious. She also seems to have some difficulty with assertiveness, and she may well be scared of conflict. All her rational responses suggest that she needs to communicate with people more clearly and assertively. This may make her anxious (she's likely to assume she won't do it well and it won't help), but trying a different strategy is likely to be quite helpful to her across a range of stressful situations in her life.

Roger, on the other hand, tends to blame other people when things go wrong. He tends to think *other* people are incompetent, inconsiderate, or lazy. As a result, Roger is often angry and frustrated. Ironically, however, he also seems to have difficulty with appropriately assertive communication. In all likelihood, Roger spends a lot of time fuming quietly, and then occasionally blows up at people when he can't take it anymore.

Not only did Amanda and Roger react to the same three situations very differently from each other, but both of them had almost the same reaction *across* the situations. Amanda ended up feeling sad and worthless, while Roger ended up feeling angry and frustrated across all three situations. Nevertheless, *both* Amanda and Roger could benefit from doing this kind of analysis, and both of them could probably also benefit from communicating more clearly with the people around them and attempting to resolve interpersonal conflict assertively and appropriately.

You may be wondering what any of this has to do with managing gut problems. Remember that *stress* has a direct effect on the ability of the gut to do its job smoothly and effectively. You can see that both Roger and Amanda are pretty stressed out a lot of the time, although in different ways and for different reasons. It's easy to imagine these situations triggering GI symptoms in both of them. Learning to think about situations more objectively and to consider the benign alternatives can help you reduce the amount of stress you experience in response to life events. Reducing your stress load will reduce your GI symptoms. I promise.

SUGGESTED ACTIVITIES

1. This week you should try to complete three of these thought records about three different situations. You can pick any situation that left you feeling the least bit stressed. It could be something relatively trivial (like a bad haircut or someone tailgating you) or something more significant (a difficult meeting at work or a fight with a loved one). Try to describe the situation as objectively as possible, without making any assumptions about other people's motivations or thoughts, underlying causes, or eventual outcomes. Next, try to identify all the relevant thoughts you had in response to the situation. Try to list all the emotions or feelings you experienced in the aftermath. Hopefully, each of the emotions will be tied to and explained by a thought. Finally, try to come up with some alternative explanations or ways of thinking about the situation that might make you feel better.

   When you've completed three thought records, read through them one after the other to look for themes in your emotional responses and your thoughts. You may or may not find any. But if you do, it's a big clue that there's something consistent about the way in which you're thinking about things that might be worth changing.

THOUGHT RECORD

SITUATION	THOUGHTS

FEELINGS	ALTERNATIVES & EVIDENCE

THOUGHT RECORD

SITUATION	THOUGHTS

FEELINGS	ALTERNATIVES & EVIDENCE

THOUGHT RECORD

SITUATION	THOUGHTS

FEELINGS	ALTERNATIVES & EVIDENCE

THOUGHT RECORD

SITUATION	THOUGHTS

FEELINGS	ALTERNATIVES & EVIDENCE

Chapter Five

APPLYING THE COGNITIVE MODEL TO GI SYMPTOMS

In the last chapter we focused on how cognitions—what we think and believe about events—can magnify stress and make us feel more upset than necessary. Hopefully, you took the time over the last week to write about a few situations in which you were able to identify your thoughts and figure out how the feelings you experienced arose directly from those thoughts. You may even have been able to come up with some *alternative* ways of thinking and to examine the evidence for each set of thoughts to determine which was most likely to be true. This week, we are going to see how some of those general skills can be applied directly to the experience of GI symptoms.

One way cognitive interventions can help with gut problems is by reducing your stress burden generally. As you've learned, the lower your general stress level, the less your GI system will be affected by the biological effects of stress and the fewer physical symptoms you should experience. But one of the unfortunate things that happens with gut problems is that not only are GI symptoms a *reaction* to stress, they are also a potential *stressor in themselves*. As with any other experience, we have beliefs and thoughts in response to the situation that can either minimize or magnify how stressful the GI symptoms themselves will be.

People have two different types of thoughts about their GI symptoms.

1. Thoughts about the physical discomfort itself. Examples include thoughts like these:

> "I can't stand this anymore."

> "I'm helpless—there's nothing I can do."

> "This is intolerable."

> "It's terrible and it's never going to get any better."

> "It's not fair."

> "If this keeps up, I'll go crazy."

2. Thoughts about the social and occupational implications of having GI symptoms. Examples include thoughts like these:

> "I won't be able to go out."

> "Even if I do go out, I won't enjoy myself."

> "I won't be able to eat or drink."

> "I'll make a fool of myself."

> "Everyone will think there's something wrong with me."

> "I'll be embarrassed or humiliated if I have to leave."

> "No one will understand."

> "People will reject me."

"I'll be fired."

"People will think I'm disgusting."

"People will think I'm weak."

"People will think I'm pathetic."

"People will think I'm crazy."

Many of these thoughts lead to intense feelings of *shame* and make people with GI problems very motivated to keep their difficulties *secret* from people around them. Somehow, gut problems just seem more disgusting, embarrassing, and humiliating than other kinds of problems—like chronic back pain or migraine headaches. As disabling as those conditions might be, they seem "cleaner" somehow, and many people believe it would be easier to let coworkers, friends, and others know about those kinds of issues than about gut problems. Unfortunately, shame and secrecy surrounding GI problems can *compound* the stress you experience enormously. If you don't feel you can explain to people around you *why* you need to stop more frequently on road trips, or limit what or where you eat, or step out of the classroom or meeting or theater, it makes things that much more difficult. Many people with gut problems make up "excuses" frequently but also worry a lot about the possible social and work-related implications of dealing with their gut issues. These beliefs—that others will be disgusted, that you will be humiliated, that you have to *hide* what's really going on at all costs—are incredibly stressful thoughts. We'll address some of these thoughts specifically in Chapter 6, "Test It Out! Behavioral Experiments." For now, you should ask yourself whether you hold these beliefs and in what ways and under what circumstances they may affect you and even limit what you do.

One way to think about all these negative thoughts surrounding GI symptoms is that they set up a *cycle* in which GI sensations lead to negative automatic thoughts, which lead to increased distress, which leads to a physical stress reaction, which increases GI symptoms. This is also known as a *vicious circle* (see below).

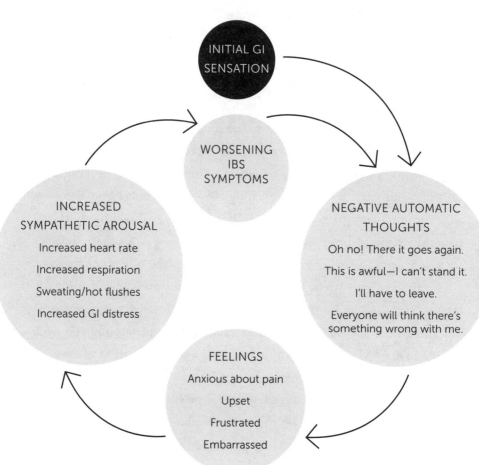

It's a *circle* because you end up back where you started—with increasing GI symptoms. It's a *vicious* circle because every time you loop around, it gets worse, and there's no obvious way out.

The good news is that you already know two places where you can intervene and stop the cycle. One place to cut the circular chain of events is here:

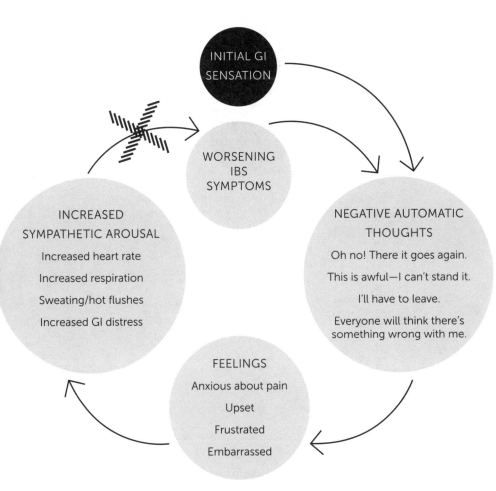

You do this with the relaxation exercises you learned in Chapter 3, "Relaxation Training." Relaxation exercises are all about reducing sympathetic nervous system arousal. Since stress leads to arousal, and arousal increases GI distress, reducing arousal using relaxation techniques should help reduce the impact of stress on your GI symptoms.

But remember, an even better way to reduce the impact of stress is to reduce the stress itself! The best way to do this is to target the negative thoughts that are making you feel stressed to begin with. That means you can intervene much earlier in the cycle:

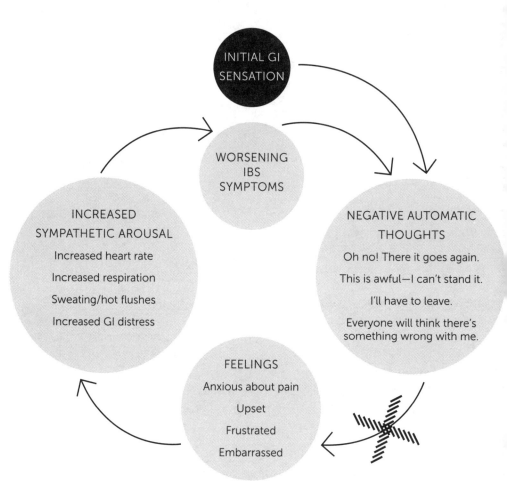

You can do this by using the same techniques you learned in Chapter 4, "The Cognitive Model of Stress Management." In this case, however, the "situation" is always going to include that you have noticed your gut starting to act up. The situation might also include some information about the context (e.g., dinner with friends, an important meeting at work, a blind date). First, you have to identify your own negative thoughts—what went through your mind when you realized your gut was starting to act up? Try this exercise now. Identify a recent episode of GI symptoms and try to remember what was going through your mind when you first noticed the symptoms. Fill in your negative automatic thoughts and the way they made you feel in the thought record below:

SITUATION (INCLUDING IBS SYMPTOMS)	THOUGHTS	FEELINGS

It's not always easy to identify our real thoughts and beliefs—especially regarding the things we are anxious or depressed about. You may be having difficulty filling in the "thoughts" part of the worksheet. One useful technique to try here is the "worst-case scenario" question. Given the situation you were in, what is the worst possible outcome that you could anticipate or imagine happening? Many people are tempted to give what they think is the "right" answer to this question—something like this: "Well, nothing would really happen. It wouldn't be a big deal." If you really believed that, you probably wouldn't be experiencing stress-related GI symptoms! Instead of giving the "right" answer, give the *real* answer. What is the worst thing you can imagine happening? People with gut problems often imagine all sorts of awful, even catastrophic outcomes. For example, people foresee all kinds of negative social and work-related outcomes, like these: "My date will think I'm weird"; "I'll have to leave the meeting and I'll be perceived as incompetent"; "I won't be able to get through the presentation"; "My friends will pity me and think I'm weak." One IBS patient I worked with even imagined that her bowels would seize up completely, she'd have to be hospitalized for some horrible procedure, and she would actually die on the table from the excruciating pain and physical damage. These are stressful thoughts! If they even cross your mind, your stress level will rise accordingly.

Now comes the challenging part. The next step is to identify some benign alternatives to the thoughts you have listed. Be careful not to simply contradict your negative predictions (e.g., by saying, "Maybe that won't happen"). The problem with such simple opposite statements is that they aren't very convincing. What you need to do is come up with an alternative scenario. For example, you might think to yourself, "If I disappear into the bathroom for a while, my date may wonder if I'm trying to ditch him. I could just tell him that there was a long line." In a work setting, you might consider the alternative that you could tolerate the gut distress for a period of time—it might calm down—and even if you do need to step out for a few minutes, no one will think that much of it as long as you present the information you are there to report.

The real key to giving these benign alternatives "teeth"—that is, making them more believable than your initial negative thoughts—is that you have to consider the *evidence* for and against each set of beliefs. For example, you might ask yourself what goes through your mind if you see someone else get up and leave a meeting for a few minutes. People often step out of meetings to go to the bathroom, refresh their coffee, take a cell phone call, and the like. Do you conclude that *they* are weird, pathetic, weak, or incompetent? Probably not! Then what evidence do you have that other people are drawing those conclusions about you? Here's another example. If you found yourself thinking, "I can't stand this," a benign alternative might be that you have, in fact, tolerated GI symptoms in the past, even in situations where it was difficult. Or perhaps you can think of other types of discomfort that you have tolerated or survived. You may well be stronger and tougher than you think. While GI discomfort certainly isn't pleasant, it's not truly catastrophic, either, especially if it's not the result of active disease. Of course you'd rather not experience those symptoms, but lots of people have to tolerate physical discomfort of all different kinds, like chronic back pain or arthritis. It's not fun. No one would choose it. But it's not the end of the world, either. It's important to start thinking of GI symptoms as *uncomfortable and annoying* rather than as *painful and disabling*. Is it fair that you have this problem? No. But it needn't be catastrophic, either.

People with Crohn's and ulcerative colitis may wonder if this same advice applies during active flare-ups. IBD flares almost always involve an increase in GI discomfort that can really only be described as painful. When I suggest downplaying that as "uncomfortable," you may feel invalidated and think I'm trivializing the very real pain you experience from time to time. Pain sucks. It's exhausting, distracting, and very, very frustrating. But here's the thing. Losing days of your life, not getting to work, missing out on time with family and friends—that sucks even more. I'm not asking you to be a superhero. There may be times when you simply need to stay home and take care of yourself. But remember, stress and distress amplify GI symptoms and, ultimately, quality of life is determined more by the activities you engage in than by your level of physical discomfort. So there may well be times when you'll be tempted to opt out of life activities, but if you go ahead and do them anyway, you'll find you can enjoy yourself and might actually feel a little bit better. A benign alternative for you might be something like this: "Well, sure, I'll be uncomfortable, but I'd rather be uncomfortable watching my daughter's concert than be uncomfortable and sad and angry that I missed it. I won't be *more* uncomfortable if I go, and I will be unhappy if I don't go."

Try this exercise now. Refer back to the scenario you wrote about above in which you identified a situation, your thoughts, and your feelings. Now enter some possible *benign alternatives* and the evidence for and against them in the thought record on the next page.

THOUGHT RECORD

SITUATION	THOUGHTS

FEELINGS	ALTERNATIVES & EVIDENCE

Coming up with benign alternatives can be particularly difficult when the automatic thoughts are reflecting deeper, more core beliefs. For example, you might be having this automatic thought: "If I have GI symptoms, it is terrible and it will ruin my day." This thought might well be based on a deeper, core belief like this: "If anything goes wrong, it ruins everything." In another example, you might think, "If I get flustered during the meeting because my gut is acting up, then everyone will think I'm an idiot." This might be based on the core belief that "If I'm not perfect, then I'm a total failure." While these extreme, black-and-white thoughts may look silly in print, it's surprising how many folks believe them without even realizing they do!

Take a moment to ask yourself whether you hold any beliefs like this. Is it truly okay for you to make a mistake or do you have trouble forgiving yourself? Does it matter if a few people don't like or respect you all that much? Is conflict intolerable to you, no matter what the situation? What if one person in a group does think you're weak, or stressed out, or weird? Is it impossible to take pleasure in an event or outing if things don't go perfectly? If you fail at one task or challenge, does that make *you* a failure? Is it unacceptable to fail?

As you learned in the last chapter, if your reactions to specific situations are driven by these kinds of core beliefs, then you have to address more than the negative automatic thoughts that are specific to the situation. You have to address the underlying core belief as well. One useful way to do this is to ask yourself what you would say to a close friend or loved one who expressed such a belief to you. Would you agree with her? Or would you argue with her? Most people hold themselves to much tougher (and more unrealistic!) standards than they hold other people. If your best friend or your child told you that he was a failure and that his life was ruined because he had screwed up one particular thing, what would you say? Now turn around and say the same thing to yourself! Why should different rules apply to you than to the rest of the people in your life? Only the gods are perfect. Real people make mistakes and have bad days. We're not liked and respected by everyone we know. A big part of this program is about learning to question extreme, unrealistic beliefs that set you up for stress and exacerbate your gut problems. If you can learn to do this, you are well on your way to conquering your IBS.

SUGGESTED ACTIVITIES

1. Continue to fill in thought records three to four times this week. Pay special attention to times when your gut is actually acting up.
2. Be sure to look for themes, watch out for core beliefs, and always to try to examine the evidence and consider things as objectively as possible.

THOUGHT RECORD

SITUATION	THOUGHTS

FEELINGS	ALTERNATIVES & EVIDENCE

THOUGHT RECORD

SITUATION	THOUGHTS

FEELINGS	ALTERNATIVES & EVIDENCE

THOUGHT RECORD

SITUATION	THOUGHTS

FEELINGS	ALTERNATIVES & EVIDENCE

THOUGHT RECORD

SITUATION	THOUGHTS

FEELINGS	ALTERNATIVES & EVIDENCE

Chapter Six

TEST IT OUT! BEHAVIORAL EXPERIMENTS

Last week I asked you to start applying the cognitive model directly to your thoughts about GI symptoms. For your homework, I asked you to complete another three to four thought records about situations in which your gut actually acted up. If you did the suggested activities, then you wrote about a few situations in which you were able to identify your thoughts, and you discovered how your thoughts about the GI symptoms themselves might actually be contributing to further stress and more symptoms. Hopefully, you were able to come up with some *alternative* ways of thinking, and to examine the *evidence* for each set of thoughts to determine which was most likely to be true.

Sometimes, however, we simply don't have enough evidence to figure out the most accurate or objective way of looking at things. We may hold beliefs without having any evidence one way or the other. For example, many people with gut problems believe that it is quite noticeable to other people when they have to excuse themselves to go to the bathroom. They don't really have any data or evidence to *support* this belief; they just assume it's true. On the other hand, when they think about it, they realize that they don't really have much data to contradict the belief, either. In other words, they just don't have enough evidence either way to decide whether that belief is accurate or not.

If you find that you hold beliefs that you can't support or contradict with evidence, then it's time to learn about *behavioral experiments*. Behavioral experiments are things you can do in the real world to gather *data* or *evidence* about beliefs. For example, suppose you are convinced that clambering over people in a row of chairs is a terrible thing to do. It's impolite, disruptive, embarrassing, and just generally not socially acceptable. Try to think of a way to gather data about this. For example, think of several different settings where people are seated in rows—the movies, a worship service, a PTA meeting, whatever. Now go to one of those settings, set yourself up where you can see most of the place, and count how many people get up at some point and clamber over other people in their row. What would you predict? That no one does it? Or do a number of people do it at some point? Now, if possible, try to gauge the reactions of the people being clambered over. Are they annoyed? Irritated? Put off? Or do people pretty much take this in stride and assume it's just a normal part of life? The results of such an experiment might surprise you.

Another approach would be to go to a movie theater, sit down, and then intentionally get up maybe half an hour into the movie and clamber over people. Go out of the theater, go back in, and sit in a different seat—climbing over people to get there. Do this again three or four times, slipping into different theaters so you're not climbing over the same people four or five times. Try to gauge the reactions of the people being climbed over. What would you predict? Would people huff and snort and roll their eyes? Or would they politely shift their legs and try to make room for you to get by? How do *you* feel if someone needs to slip past you in a row of seats? What do you conclude about that person? If your beliefs about other people are basically benign, why do you think other people have negative beliefs about you?

Good behavioral experiments have several components, just like good scientific experiments. First, you have to have a hypothesis, a belief that you are putting to the test. Second, you need to set up a situation in which you can actually test the belief. Third, you have to have predictions about what will happen if the belief is true, as opposed to what will happen if the belief is not true. Fourth, you have to go do the experiment and pay attention to what *actually* happens. Finally, you have to compare your prediction (what you thought would happen if your belief were true) to what actually happened (which may suggest that your original belief needs to be modified or changed).

For example, many people with gut problems believe that their friends would be grossed out, or would think they were weird or pathetic, if they knew about their "bathroom" issues. It's not hard to set up a situation in which you can test this belief. Identify a close friend, someone you like and basically trust, who doesn't know about your gut problems, and explain to him or her a little bit about the difficulties you've been having. If your belief were true, you would *predict* that your friend would react in an awkward or unpleasant way. Perhaps at best he or she might change the subject very quickly without expressing much sympathy or concern or even curiosity. If your belief were *not* true, you would predict that your friend would react quite differently—expressing interest and concern and sympathy.

Now you have to go and tell your friend, and pay attention to how he or she *actually* reacts. This may feel very scary. You're taking a risk here. If your friend reacts well—that's great. You can start modifying your upsetting belief. But if your belief is true, and your friend reacts awkwardly or unpleasantly, you're stuck with having told him or her. So ask yourself—what would be the worst thing about that? Maybe your friend reacted awkwardly because he or she just didn't know what to say. Maybe his or her opinion of you has actually changed—and for the worse. If that's the case, is this someone you *really* want to remain friends with? Good friends are understanding. Most people are sympathetic and flexible and just add new information to enrich their knowledge of someone. In the vast majority of cases, people feel *honored* to be taken into someone's confidence. It makes them feel closer to you because they know you trust them. Many people will eventually return the honor by sharing more personal information about themselves with you. That's how friendships grow and deepen. So, while it's true that you might be taking a risk by carrying out this sort of behavioral experiment, you are also opening yourself up to the possibility of greater intimacy, trust, and confidence in a friendship. If it doesn't work out—if the person you choose turns out to be unsympathetic, or laughs at you, or is mean about it—you have a problem to solve; you need to find a better friend!

This exercise may be particularly anxiety-provoking if you harbor a great deal of *shame* about your GI issues and have been working hard to keep your gut problems *secret*. Do you frequently make up excuses for having to skip social or work events involving food and drink? Do you worry a lot about what clients or coworkers or your boss or even friends and family will think about your using the bathroom frequently? Why? What are the underlying assumptions you're making here about how people would react if they knew the truth? Chances are, you're assuming that people would respond *much* more negatively than they actually would. If you present your condition in a straightforward, matter-of-fact way, people will generally take it in stride. Most people will be somewhat interested, genuinely concerned, flattered that you told them, and relieved that there isn't something else going on, like that you don't really like them all that much and that's why you won't meet them for drinks or dinner. Remember that other people catastrophize too!

I could share many examples from patients' lives about when they finally got up the nerve to share the basics about their GI condition with someone and discovered, to their intense relief, that the person was pleased to know, thought better of them for having been straightforward, and worked with them to accommodate their need for more frequent bathroom visits. One businessman, who had to travel frequently for work, came up with an endless variety of "I must have had a bad burrito" stories to explain why he couldn't join his colleagues at restaurants or in the hotel bar after the day's work. He finally learned that telling people he had a chronic GI condition and wouldn't be drinking, but would be happy to hang out for an hour after the meeting was met with polite interest and occasional curiosity, and that most people simply said, "Glad you told me. See you at the bar!" One of my favorites is from a woman with Crohn's who was working in a rehabilitation health care setting. She ended up telling her supervisor, and they agreed to let patients know, very briefly and appropriately, that she might need to step out on occasion because of a GI-related medical issue of her own. To her delight and surprise, not only were her coworkers supportive, but many of her patients told her how *inspired* they were by her. They saw her as professional and effective, and it gave them hope that they could overcome their own medical issues and live an equally satisfying life.

So if you are one of those people who has been keeping your GI issues secret from people around you, now is the time to try a behavioral experiment to see what would really happen if you just told people. Don't make a big deal of it. It doesn't have to be a dramatic revelation. Just pick someone you feel reasonably comfortable with and, when you have an opportunity, let him or her know that you have a chronic GI condition that sometimes causes gut upset, and that you occasionally have to watch what you eat and/or make more frequent bathroom trips. Some people won't want to know any more. Many people may be curious and they *may* want to know more. Tell them as much as you feel comfortable revealing. Keep it light, factual, and straightforward. If it feels right, use humor. Acknowledge that sometimes it's frustrating or limiting, but you make the best of it and don't let it interfere with life. Then pay attention to how they react. Did any of your dire predictions come true? Or did the person react kindly and genuinely? You might very well be pleasantly surprised!

To summarize, in a behavioral experiment you want to:

1. **Identify** the negative belief you *want* to test and think of relevant situations you could set up that would let you test the belief.

2. **Predict** what will happen if the belief is true and consider what might happen if the belief is not true.

3. **Gather data** by carrying out the experiment and pay attention to what *actually* happens, even if this feels scary or seems to entail some risk.

4. **Compare** what actually happened with what you predicted. What does the evidence suggest about your original belief?

Another example of a behavioral experiment is to test the belief that if you feel a sudden urge to defecate, you *must* get to a bathroom or something catastrophic will happen. Interestingly, lots of biological urges actually go away temporarily even if you don't satisfy them. This includes hunger; sleepiness; cravings for drugs, including caffeine and nicotine; and the urge to defecate. Obviously, you have to respond to some of these urges eventually. You certainly can't go indefinitely without eating, sleeping, or defecating. But you *can* delay responding to them without undue stress. In most cases, the urge will peak and then recede for a while. Remember that the colon is *designed* to hold onto stool until there's a convenient place to go. If you are one of the many people with IBS who are convinced that they always have to be within thirty seconds of a bathroom, you might want to try the following experiment. At home, where it's safe and the consequences are very small, try delaying defecating by a minute or two, at first, when you have a sudden urge and see what happens. You might just find that the urge subsides. You can slowly build up the time between the initial urge and the time you defecate. If the urge does subside, you can simply wait for the next urge to hit and then go to the bathroom. The more you convince yourself that you *can* "hold it," the less important it will seem to know where the bathrooms are and the less scary it will be when a bathroom might be tough to get to quickly (car trips, bus rides, and so on).

If you're having an IBD flare, you will have to modify these exercises somewhat, but it doesn't mean you can't do them. Behavioral medicine experts have known for years that some people with chronic diseases are quite disabled by them, while other people *with equal disease severity* seem to live fuller, happier lives. What's the difference? It isn't that the people in that second group are somehow "tougher" or "stronger" or have higher pain tolerance. It's that they choose to live fully despite having some limitations. So, for example, if you would normally avoid going shopping or to a theater during a flare, go anyway, even if you do end up sitting in the back by the aisle and scoping out the bathrooms first. If that's what it takes to get you out the door, then do it and *go*! Bring a change of underwear if you must, but don't miss out on life.

Remember that the purpose of all the cognitive work I introduced you to in Chapter 4, "The Cognitive Model of Stress Management," and Chapter 5, "Applying the Cognitive Model to GI Symptoms," was *not* for you to put rose-colored glasses on. I don't want you to trade in a depressing or anxiety-provoking worldview for a falsely optimistic worldview. What I want is for you to be able to evaluate your beliefs *objectively* in light of the evidence. Recall the very first hypothetical example of waving to your friend across the street (see page 53). If you just try to tell yourself, "He or she didn't see me," without any evidence (or even contrary to the evidence that the last time you spoke you had a fight), then the cognitive interventions aren't going to be very convincing!

The problem with cognitive interventions alone is that lots of times we just don't have the evidence we need to know whether our initial negative beliefs are right or not. We may be able to come up with benign alternatives, but without the evidence to convince us, those may not help much. That's where behavioral experiments come in. They are clever ways of gathering data to help us decide which beliefs are valid and which ones aren't. Sometimes a behavioral experiment can be as simple as asking someone what he or she thinks. Of course, you have to trust that he or she will tell you the truth, and you have to be a little cautious about asking some people certain things. For example, I wouldn't necessarily ask my CEO if farting at meetings is problematic. But I might ask a trusted family member or very close friend how much they actually notice my farting and how much they care. If he or she knows you want to hear the truth, he or she will probably tell you.

Other times behavioral experiments have to be more subtle or more clever, or you may have to set up situations that will allow you to test certain beliefs. Sometimes you can gather data about other people just by watching them, as in the movie theater example, in which you simply count the number of times other people get up and clamber over others during a movie.

Sometimes behavioral experiments can feel very scary. It's always a good idea to initially pick something that feels doable, so that even if the outcome isn't what you hoped for (your boyfriend tells you that he does notice your farts and doesn't exactly think they're cute), you still have someplace positive to go with it (after all, he loves you anyway and isn't going anywhere, so maybe it doesn't matter all that much). The more you can incorporate behavioral experiments into your life, the less likely it is that unfounded negative thoughts will continue to control your emotional life and the better off you will be.

SUGGESTED ACTIVITIES

1. Try to think of one behavioral experiment you could do this week that would provide some real data about a negative belief you hold and go do it.

2. Continue to do thought records two to three times a week. The situations don't have to be "big"—anything that caused you the least twinge of stress or anxiety will work. The point is to keep practicing these skills until they become second nature.

Chapter Seven
ELIMINATING AVOIDANCE

This week, we're going to switch gears and start talking about *avoidance*—something lots of people with gut problems are very good at!

Avoidance is a perfectly natural and often adaptive coping strategy. In fact, if we didn't learn to avoid things that were bad for us, we wouldn't live very long! The first time you get a burn, you learn to *avoid* touching hot things. If you know something is dangerous, you *should* avoid it! Unfortunately, humans often avoid things for the wrong reasons, and avoiding things you don't really need to avoid is usually a pretty bad idea.

Here are some examples of common but maladaptive avoidance behaviors.

1. **Procrastination.** People often avoid doing things because they are anxious about them. They think things like "I hate this. It's overwhelming. It will be too hard or too unpleasant. I won't be able to do it. It'll feel awful. I'll be bad at it. Even if I do it, it'll turn out badly." Sound familiar? Everyone procrastinates sometimes. The problem with procrastination, of course, is that it actually makes you feel worse. Now you still have the task to do, and you feel guilty and even more anxious on top

of it because you let it go too long. Most of the time, once we actually sit ourselves down to do the task, it turns out to be much easier and less painful than we were anticipating. One useful trick is to make a deal with yourself—sit down and work on it for five to ten minutes. If it really feels awful, you can stop. In the vast majority of cases, you find it's really not that bad, and you just keep working!

2. **Phobic avoidance.** People with phobias of specific things (like elevators or dogs or spiders) often go to great lengths to avoid coming into contact with the thing they're scared of. It can get to the point where it actually interferes with life. The problem with avoidance is that people never have the chance to learn that the thing they're so scared of really isn't that dangerous.

3. **Social avoidance.** This is a big one for a lot of people. In some people, this is severe enough to be diagnosed as social anxiety disorder. But *lots* of people have mild social avoidance. Maybe they hate speaking up in class or in meetings. Maybe they have to have a drink or two every time they go to a party just to tolerate being there. Clearly, this could get in your way professionally or socially. What's less obvious is that avoidance actually makes anxiety *worse*. You become more and more convinced that you *can't* do the things you avoid doing. As a result, they get scarier and scarier, and you never have the chance to learn new skills or to realize that you actually can do these things.

People with gut problems typically avoid a number of things for reasons that *look* perfectly sensible on the face of them. The problem with this is twofold. First, it can really limit your life and make things less fun and less productive. Second, it may actually be making your gut problems *worse*. Once you start avoiding a few things, it gets more and more tempting to avoid lots of things. If you have started to avoid things because of your GI symptoms, you probably already know that this isn't working out that well for you. You may have escaped or avoided a few stressful things in the short run, but in the long run, your life isn't better because you're avoiding things. It's worse. The bottom line is that

AVOIDANCE DOESN'T WORK

Here's a list of the sorts of things people with gut problems often avoid.

VISCERAL SENSATIONS

Most people with gut problems are both hypersensitive to visceral (or gut) sensations and hypervigilant about them. Because they fear the onset of GI symptoms, they monitor their bodies for signs of an impending attack. People with IBS often go to great lengths to avoid experiencing those sensations, if at all possible. They view abdominal discomfort as intolerable—painful, debilitating, incapacitating—and something to be avoided by whatever means necessary. This leads to avoidance of lots of other things (tight clothing that presses on the belly, possible "trigger" foods, and stressful situations), and to the use of medications (like antidiarrheal drugs), in a futile attempt to fend off any and all abdominal discomfort. It also leads to retreating from life experiences, opportunities, and challenges (in favor of, say, curling up in bed with a heating pad pressed to the tummy).

One of the most important things you can do to help yourself overcome the disabling aspects of IBS is to stop thinking of GI symptoms as painful attacks that make you sick and must be avoided at all costs, and start thinking about them as uncomfortable, annoying, occasionally inconvenient, but not catastrophic. *Everyone* experiences uncomfortable visceral sensations from time to time. Yours are undoubtedly somewhat worse and somewhat more frequent, which isn't fair or fun, but they're not catastrophic, either. It's unrealistic to try to avoid visceral sensations altogether. But if you can learn that not all twinges, cramps, or gurgles are dangerous, and many visceral sensations can be acknowledged and then safely ignored (like the smoke detector that goes off every time you boil water), you'll be well on your way to taking back control of your life.

Of course, if you have an IBD and are in the middle of an active flare, then you may *need* to track your symptoms and be in touch with your doctor. Sometimes abdominal pain can signal a condition (like a small bowel obstruction) that really *does* need medical attention. In severe IBD, such things could even require emergency intervention. The key for people with IBDs is to learn to tell the difference between sensations that signal a real problem and sensations that can safely be ignored. If you've experienced true medical emergencies with IBD, you are especially likely to be hypervigilant about abdominal discomfort. The more objective you can be about understanding different sensations and levels of discomfort, and learning which ones are important and which ones probably aren't, the better off you'll be. Talk to your physician about when it is important to seek medical attention, and when you can safely ignore or delay attending to visceral sensations.

FOODS

People with gut problems develop all kinds of beliefs about which foods do or do not upset them. In fact, many IBS websites have lists of "danger" or "trigger" foods that they insist people with IBS should avoid at all costs. Some of the most commonly cited "no-no" foods and drinks include coffee; dairy; meat; wheat; fruit; fried, greasy, or spicy foods; carbonated beverages; chocolate; alcohol; salad greens and raw veggies; and legumes like beans. Much of the same advice is often given to people with Crohn's, with very little or no supporting evidence. People with Crohn's may have to make dietary changes during acute flares, but there is very little data suggesting that those changes need to be maintained when they're not having an active flare. There's no question that different foods affect digestive processes differently. (See Chapter 8, "Diet and IBS," for a detailed discussion of diet.) But people sometimes elevate food avoidance to an art form! They develop all kinds of complicated strategies and rules for managing food to the point where it becomes difficult to keep track of it all, and some or most of it may not be necessary or even helpful. Moreover, sometimes people get so anxious about whether a food might upset them that they develop *superstitious* avoidance. Say you once ate a hamburger, and later that night or even the next day your gut acted up. You might conclude you should never eat hamburgers again. But what if your gut acted up for totally different reasons—say, because you had a stressful meeting coming up? Then you're denying yourself hamburgers for no good reason! If you have been avoiding or severely limiting a number of foods, you need to read Chapter 8, which covers the scientific evidence about diet. But before you read Chapter 8, take a moment to reflect on what you currently believe about food and your GI symptoms, and list foods you typically avoid or restrict.

MY BELIEFS ABOUT FOOD

FOODS I AVOID OR RESTRICT

SITUATIONS INVOLVING FOOD

Another category of things people with gut problems often prefer to avoid are *situations* that are likely to involve food and eating. This obviously includes restaurants, but it also includes parties, being invited to people's homes, social events at bars or clubs, any place where there is likely to be social eating and/or drinking, and where it might be awkward or embarrassing to refuse certain foods, ask for special foods, or have gut problems related to particular foods.

In the box below, go ahead and list any food-related situations you might tend to avoid. Note if you always avoid them, sometimes avoid them, occasionally avoid them, or wish you could avoid them altogether, even though you don't.

FOOD SITUATIONS I PREFER TO AVOID

SITUATIONS WHERE BATHROOMS ARE HARD TO FIND

People with gut problems often prefer to avoid situations in which they might get stuck in some way, especially places where it might be hard to get to a bathroom, or where others would notice if they got up and left. Common situations that people with GI symptoms tend to avoid include the following:

Situations related to transportation:

Long car trip   Airplane

Subway   Elevator

Train   Bridge/Tunnel

Bus

Situations in which many people sit in rows:

Places of worship	Sports stadiums
Movie theaters	Classes
Concerts or shows	

Crowded public places or places where you might get stuck in line:

Shopping malls	Zoos
Supermarkets	Amusement parks

Places or situations where bathrooms are hard to find or hard to get to:

Beach	Parks
Camping	Outdoor concerts or events
Skiing	

Work situations in which leaving might be difficult:

Meetings	Conference calls
Conferences	Front desk/Reception
Presentations	

In the box on the next page, please list the places or situations you generally prefer to avoid. If you hardly avoid anything, good for you! Just note that you don't avoid things. If you do avoid things, do your best to list the situations *in order of difficulty* for you. That is, first list the places you would always avoid, if possible, or tolerate only with extreme difficulty, then go down in difficulty until you get to places you'd sometimes prefer to avoid, but can tolerate fairly well, even on a bad day. Next to each place or situation, I'd also like you to rate how much distress you think it would cause you if you had to be there. Use a scale from 0 to 100, where 100 is horrendous, intolerable anxiety, stress, and upset—the worst you've ever experienced; 60 or 70 is awful—really hard to tolerate, although you could suck it up for a very short period of time; 40 or 50 is pretty bad; 20 or 30 isn't much fun, but you could definitely tolerate it if you had to; 10 is just a bit of discomfort, "normal" anxiety, or a tiny bit of gut distress. This is called a *subjective unit of distress* (or SUD) score. There's nothing magical about it. You could rate things from 1 to 10, or 0 to 7, or according to whatever scale you want. We usually use 0 to 100 because it provides lots of ratings in the middle of the scale. Do your best to order the things on your list so that the distress rating starts really high and goes down pretty low, with a few things in the middle of the rating scale as well. Also be sure you have some items that are very low on the list, things you could do with only minimal discomfort.

SITUATIONS I PREFER TO AVOID	SUD SCORE
Things it would be *extremely* difficult or even impossible for me to do:	80–100
Things it would be *quite* difficult to tolerate:	60–79
Things it would be *moderately* difficult to do:	40–59

SITUATIONS I PREFER TO AVOID	SUD SCORE
Things I could do that would be *uncomfortable* but bearable:	20–39
Things I could do with only *minimal* discomfort or anxiety:	0–19

SUBTLE AVOIDANCE

The last category of things people with gut problems often avoid may not sound like avoidance to you at all. I call this category *subtle avoidance* because, while it looks like you're engaging in activities and going places, you're really still doing things to avoid the *possibility* of embarrassment, discomfort, or distress related to GI symptoms. One thing people with gut problems often do is scope out any new place to be sure they know where the bathrooms are. Another thing people with IBS do is place themselves strategically so that they can make a quick exit, or get to the bathroom quickly, or leave the place or situation unobtrusively. Examples of this include sitting at the back of a room where others can't see you, sitting at the end of an aisle or pew so you don't have to clamber over people, and sitting near a window or door or anywhere you think will make you feel less anxious. Some people with IBS will take a swig of an antigas or anti-diarrheal medication like Maalox® or Pepto-Bismol or Imodium before going out. Others carry around a prescription medication like Lomotil with them. They may never even use any of it, but just having it with them makes them feel more secure. If you engage in these or any other "subtle" avoidance behaviors, please list them below. As you did above, try to list them in order, so that the things that would be most anxiety-provoking to give up are listed at the top, and things that are the least important to you, or would be the least difficult to give up, are listed at the bottom. Be sure to give each one a SUD score that represents the degree of distress you think you'd experience if you tried to give up that behavior.

SITUATIONS I PREFER TO AVOID	SUD SCORE
Things it would be *extremely* difficult or even impossible for me to give up:	80–100
Things it would be *quite* difficult to give up:	60–79
Things it would be *moderately* difficult to give up:	40–59

SITUATIONS I PREFER TO AVOID	SUD SCORE
Things I could give up that would feel *uncomfortable* but bearable:	20–39
Things I could give up with only *minimal* discomfort or anxiety:	0–19

Now, let's acknowledge that when you've been avoiding things, it's no good at all for someone to tell you to "just do it." Your friends and family may have tried this, in which case you know it isn't helpful. In fact, it can actually make things worse. Here's how it often unfolds. Imagine that you force yourself to "suck it up" and try going somewhere or doing something that makes you really anxious. Maybe you can endure it for a short time, but it gets overwhelming and you leave. Or you endure it for a while and your gut acts up so much that you have an awful experience. Either way, you've basically confirmed that it was awful and that you probably *should* have avoided it in the first place. You may even be *more* anxious about it from now on. Not good! And definitely not what we're going for here. You need some other strategy to help you overcome avoidance.

If you are avoiding situations or places, it's time to learn about *exposure therapy*. Exposure therapy is based on some very straightforward principles of learning, and there is *tons* of evidence that it works. The basic logic behind exposure therapy is that you have to expose yourself *slowly* to whatever you're afraid of. When you carve things up into little, manageable chunks, it's much easier to do them. Approaching the problem of avoidance this way is much gentler and much more likely to be successful. Eventually, exposure therapy lets you handle things that would be awful for you if you tried them right away with minimal discomfort and anxiety. Let's look at a fairly straightforward example of exposure therapy in action with a very specific problem—fear of snakes.

Imagine for a moment that you are really creeped out by snakes. (This probably won't be hard. Most people in the world really don't like snakes much. In fact, most *primates* really don't like snakes much!) But now imagine that your fear of snakes is so bad that it interferes with your life. You won't go camping or even do any gardening because you might encounter a snake. You freak out if a snake appears on TV or in a movie, or if you come across a picture of a snake in a magazine. What would you normally do? Avoid them! Even to the point of quickly changing the channel or closing the magazine. What does that avoidance do? It sensitizes you! You see the picture or image, your heart thuds, you feel a little jolt of adrenaline, you quickly get rid of the image, and then you start to feel less scared. You've just told your brain, "Wow! That was scary and dangerous! Good thing I got away from it." This seems to confirm that snakes are really threatening and should be avoided at all costs.

In exposure therapy, the first thing we do is construct an *anxiety hierarchy*. This is just a fancy term for a list of things that scare you, from most scary to least scary. The scariest thing for a snake-phobic person would probably be trying to wrap a live snake around his or her neck. The least scary thing might be looking at a small picture of a very young, harmless snake. There would probably be lots of things in the middle, including looking at a snake in a glass cage at the zoo, putting a hand up to the glass of the cage, taking the lid off the cage of a harmless pet snake, touching the snake with one finger while the snake was being held by someone else, and so on. Each of these things could be rated on a scale from 0 to 100 in terms of how scary or anxiety-provoking it would be.

The next step would be for you to *expose* yourself to the lowest-ranked thing on the hierarchy. This might be a benign picture of a little baby garden snake. It might cause about 20 SUD units of anxiety. The trick is—and this is important—that you would need to *keep looking* at the picture until your discomfort began to go away. This is technically called *habituation*. But it basically means that your brain gets bored of the stimulus. You can stare at a picture only for so long without realizing that nothing bad is actually happening. It might take five minutes, or twenty minutes, but eventually the picture just stops being scary, and your SUD rating drops to between 0 and 5.

Now here's the beautiful part. The *next* thing on the hierarchy, say walking into a room with a caged snake fifteen feet away, might originally have been about a 30 or 35 on the anxiety hierarchy. But once the picture no longer feels scary to you, walking into the room feels like only about a 20 on the SUD scale. Sure, your anxiety level goes back up, but not as high as it would have if walking into the room was the first thing you had done. Again, you just have to sit by the door until your discomfort begins to subside. Snakes are actually pretty boring. They just lie under a log almost all the time. Watching a snake in a cage is a lot like watching paint drying. Booorrring! So, eventually, your brain stops sending "DANGER!" signals and gets the message that nothing much is really going on here. You've learned that this isn't so terrible, you can handle the distress, and you don't need to avoid this level of contact with snakes after all.

And, like magic, the next thing on the list drops down in terms of how anxiety-provoking it will feel. It's as if you had a stack of wooden blocks, and every time you pull one out from the bottom, the higher ones all drop down a level too. This goes on, step by step, until eventually you find that you have worked your way all the way up to the top of the hierarchy. But the amazing thing is that by the time you actually pick up the snake yourself, it causes only about 25 to 30 SUD units of anxiety. If you had tried that right off the bat, it would have been up at 100, and you wouldn't have been able to tolerate it. People sometimes mistakenly think that the goal of exposure therapy is to get them to tolerate extreme distress. Nothing could be further from the truth. When done well, exposure therapy *never* results in discomfort much higher than about a 30 on your SUD scale. Not much fun, perhaps, but certainly tolerable, especially since it tends to come down pretty quickly.

Now, the good news is that you've already done the first step—you created your anxiety hierarchies earlier in this chapter. Hopefully this was useful in and of itself. Just creating the anxiety hierarchy often helps people realize that not all situations are equally horrible or difficult to tolerate. Sometimes when we're anxious, we tend to lump all related situations into one big, scary, undoable blob. Teasing that blob apart into more- and less-anxiety-provoking steps helps you realize that you can probably do more than you might think.

Your homework this week is to focus on two situations that you avoid or prefer to avoid, or two examples of subtle avoidance. Pick two of the easiest things—ones that are the lowest on your SUD scale, preferably not more than about 25 units of distress—and *go do them*. Depending on how avoidant you tend to be, it might be something as small as "drive around the block a bunch of times" or as big as "take the train into the city." The key is to make sure you do it long enough for your anxiety to come down from a high of about 25 to at most a 10, or better yet 5 or even 0. As long as your anxiety is on the way *down*, you can stop doing it. If the thing involves an activity (like driving) or a situation (like a restaurant), be sure you stick with it long enough for the anxiety to begin to come down. For example, if you really hate being "stuck" in a car, drive around the block ten or fifteen times. That way, you're always close to home (which makes it a lot less anxiety-provoking), but you stick with it long enough for it to get boring.

I *don't* want you to pick something too hard. It's especially important to stick with whatever you choose until the anxiety begins to come down.

If you abandon ship while the anxiety is still up or, worse yet, still rising, you might sensitize yourself. This shouldn't be a big, scary thing. Just something small that you can imagine doing with some discomfort but can certainly imagine tolerating. (Sensitization isn't the end of the world—it can be fixed by going lower on the hierarchy and starting over. So don't sweat this too much.)

For example, if getting on a commuter train (the kind with no bathrooms onboard) feels too scary, just go to the train station and hang out for an hour. This may sound utterly ridiculous to you, but you're teaching your brain to stop associating riding trains with heightened anxiety, fear, and danger. The next time you go, stand around on the platform for an hour, but don't board a train. Sit on a bench. Watch people come and go. Familiarize yourself with the rhythms of the station. This will get boring pretty quickly. The next time you go, board a train, go one stop, and then get off again. Wait for the next train going back toward home, board it, and go back home. Depending on the time of day, this may take a while, and you'll probably be pretty bored by the time you get home. That's good! Boredom is like the opposite of fear. The next time you go, plan to ride the train for two or three stops. If you're feeling just fine, go all the way to some final destination that interests you. Then turn around and come home. The point is to realize that any task or situation that you have typically avoided and that feels challenging or anxiety-provoking can be broken up into smaller pieces that feel quite doable.

Note that you may experience some physical discomfort just as a result of the anxiety itself. You may be gassy or feel your gut cramping a bit, even if you haven't eaten any of your trigger foods. What we're mostly focused on here is the anxiety that goes with those sensations, not the sensations themselves. That is, one of the things you must keep in mind is that GI distress is annoying and uncomfortable, not catastrophic and life-limiting. In other words, one of the things you may need to expose yourself to is GI distress itself! That may sound a little crazy to you—after all, the whole reason you're reading this is that you want to experience far less GI distress. Remember the lessons of last week, however—sometimes people with gut problems get so anxious about the very idea of experiencing GI symptoms that their gut distress becomes this huge, life-altering, scary thing in and of itself. That's why subtle avoidance is so tricky to deal with—it's all about avoiding the perceived terrible consequences of having GI symptoms.

Obviously, if your doctor has told you to avoid specific foods, don't use those foods in this exercise. Moreover, if a certain food *always* predictably upsets your gut or gives you gas, don't eat it. If you have an IBD and are having an active flare, then you should absolutely follow your doctor's advice about limiting or avoiding foods that might be medically problematic (e.g., avoiding high-residue foods like celery or popcorn if you have a partial stricture). But if there are foods that you have been avoiding because you've heard or have read that they are "danger" foods, it's probably a good idea to expose yourself to a little bit of the food and see what happens. The point of exposure therapy should be to reduce your anxiety in specific situations or environments in which you often or usually feel somewhat anxious. It's far more important to be able to *go* to a restaurant with friends than it is to try to force yourself to eat greasy French fries or drink coffee. But if you are *afraid* of food, that very fear may be exacerbating your gut distress. Avoiding food is such an important topic for people with IBS that I've devoted an entire chapter to it. If you're one of those people who restricts your diet a great deal and consistently avoids a wide array of foods because you believe they're "dangerous triggers," read Chapter 8, "Diet and IBS," and then think about some exposure exercises you might try to address these issues.

In the text box on the next page, please write down the two things you're going to try to do this week. I'd also like you to record your predictions about what you think will happen. When you try each of the things, you'll need to record what actually happens, including how uncomfortable you got and how long it took for the discomfort or anxiety level to come down again.

EXPOSURE EXERCISES I CAN TRY	PREDICTIONS How uncomfortable will I get? How long will it last?	RESULTS How uncomfortable did I get? How long did it last?

TROUBLESHOOTING

If you find that you're having difficulty even getting yourself to do this assignment, see if you can identify the thoughts behind it. What is the worst thing that could happen? Would it be truly catastrophic? Do you see the point in trying to stop avoiding things? Most people with IBS resent the perceived need to avoid things. They just don't see the point in pushing themselves to do things that might make them uncomfortable. Hopefully, you're at the point by now where you understand that visceral discomfort isn't the end of the world, that in the vast majority of cases the "worst-case" scenario doesn't come to pass, and that even if it *does*, it may not be as bad as you once feared. The point of exposure therapy is to help you *reclaim your life*. It *works* and is a central part of every effective intervention for IBS that has been developed. So if you've been hesitant to try it, do yourself a favor. Pick something really small and easy to do and *give it a shot*. Think of this as a behavioral experiment. You may think exposure is pointless or won't work. But if you've never tried it, you really don't *know* that that's true. Thousands of scientific studies have proven the efficacy of exposure therapy and dozens of studies have applied exposure therapy *specifically* to IBS. It works. You just have to prove it to yourself.

Keep in mind that lots of different kinds of things can happen when people first start trying exposure therapy. If you tried it but had difficulty with the assignment, or you found that the anxiety did not come down, then you probably tried to do something too hard. The key to exposure therapy is to start small and *stick with it*. For example, suppose you decided to try to take the commuter train into town. You anticipated it would raise your SUD score to about 25. But when you got on the train, your SUD score shot up to 40 or 50, and you ended up getting off at the next stop. Next time, just go to the train station and hang out with a good book or a magazine for an hour. Don't even get on a train! The idea is to sneak up on the things that make you anxious, and to do it in a way that lets you associate those things with feeling calm, relaxed, even bored, rather than anxious. Once being in the train station itself is just boring, then it may be time to get on a train. But plan to go only one stop. Then get off. Then get back on and go one more stop. Then get off. Keep doing this until that in itself gets boring. (It may also be time-consuming, depending on the time of day and the train schedule.)

Another difficulty people have is that they don't stick with an activity long enough. Suppose you make yourself go to the supermarket to buy a few items and wait in line. You might get through it by going through the express line and getting out of there as fast as possible, but chances are your anxiety will still be up when you leave. The goal should be to go to the supermarket and just hang out until you get bored. The first day, you might sit in your car in the parking lot for an hour. I know this may sound absurd, but remember that we want to set you up for success. You want to pick something to do that is predictably boring and doable and that won't arouse too much distress. The next day you might walk around the supermarket for half an hour at a fairly slow time of day without even buying anything. (Put a basket over your arm and read a lot of labels so you don't feel goofy.) The point is to stick with it until your anxiety level begins to come down.

Oftentimes, people have the opposite problem with exposure therapy—the first thing they try doesn't make them anxious *enough*! It ends up being much easier and less anxiety-provoking or uncomfortable than they predicted. That's actually a fine way to start. Just be sure that you progress to the next thing up on the hierarchy. Exposure therapy helps only if you are tackling things that are at least a little bit anxiety-provoking.

The other thing to remember about exposure therapy is that it isn't a one-shot cure. You have to keep doing it, slowly working your way up your anxiety hierarchy. We usually suggest that people practice something on their list *every day*. You can do the same thing a few days in a row. You should find that you don't get as anxious the second day as you did the first day, and the anxiety should come down even faster. After a few days, you should try the next thing on your list.

It's also important to target any types of subtle avoidance you engage in. Lots of times people who engage in subtle avoidance don't even end up "needing" the thing they do. That is, you may scope out the locations of bathrooms, and then, most of the time, you find you don't need them. Even if you did need to find a bathroom, you don't necessarily need to know in advance where it is located. For most people, even people with IBS, a *feeling* of urgency doesn't mean you *actually* have to get to a bathroom instantly. You can take the time to ask where the restroom is. Ironically, trying to stop subtle avoidance behaviors is sometimes the most difficult thing to convince yourself to do. It may seem perfectly rational to carry a powerful, quick-acting antidiarrheal medication like Lomotil with you when you're out and about. You may question why you should even try to target that. Medications like Imodium and Lomotil are very effective antidiarrheal agents. They typically have a benign side effect profile (except for the pesky problem of constipation) and they don't cause addiction in any way. So why not use them? (Note: For people with an IBD, these exercises do not apply to medications that have been pre-scribed by your doctor to target the underlying disease process and man-age symptoms during active flares. Always follow your doctor's medical advice when it comes to treatment for IBD.)

The reason to leave the Lomotil at home, or to sit in the middle of a row of seats, or to go shopping without consulting a bathroom-finder website, is that these things are all part of a pattern of thoughts and behaviors that keeps your gut in control of your life. Every time you check that the Lomotil is in your purse or briefcase or glove compart-ment, you cede a bit more ground to IBS. "Gut distress is intolerable and must be avoided at all costs" is the message you send your brain. So try leaving the Lomotil at home. Go ahead and sit in the middle of the row. Go to the mall without immediately scoping out where the nearest restroom is. By sending your brain the message that you can do these things safely, you help reduce the sense of danger people with gut problems often experience. *You* have the power to turn your GI problems from an ever-present, disabling condition to a minor, slightly annoying inconvenience that doesn't really impact your quality of life all that much. And that's what this program is all about.

SUGGESTED ACTIVITIES

1. If you can identify any avoidance behaviors you engage in, try to do at least two or three exposure therapy exercises over the course of the week. Be sure to pick something that feels doable to start with, but also try to work your way up to something that felt harder initially.

Chapter Eight

DIET AND IBS

Because of media hype and woefully inadequate information, too many people nowadays are deathly afraid of their food, and what does fear of food do to the digestive system? I am sure that an unhappy or suspicious stomach, constricted and uneasy with worry, cannot digest properly. And if digestion is poor, the whole body politic suffers.

—Julia Child, *The Way to Cook*

One of the biggest myths about IBS is that there is an ideal IBS diet that will reduce or resolve symptoms for most or all IBS sufferers. You will see all kinds of recommendations out there, in books, on the web, and even in the research literature. Eat a high-fiber diet. Eat a low-fiber diet. Eat only the right kind of fiber. Avoid all milk products with lactose and switch to soy products instead. Avoid soy products at all costs. Avoid wheat and gluten. Avoid eggs. Avoid meat and follow a vegetarian diet. Avoid raw vegetables, beans, and fruit. Eat a diet very low in carbohydrates. Avoid spicy food. Avoid greasy food. Avoid fat altogether. Take probiotics or mint or ginger. Don't take mint or ginger. If you tried to follow *all* the advice out there about "trigger" foods, you'd end up with nothing at all on your plate except a pile of plain white rice and a lactobacillus pill. Not a very appetizing, nutritious, or practical solution.

The reason for all this conflicting advice is that different people with IBS respond differently to different foods. A diet that works well for a person with constipation-predominant IBS (e.g., one high in wheat bran) might be disastrous for a person with diarrhea-predominant IBS. That seems fairly obvious. What is less obvious is that a diet that works wonders for one person with diarrhea-predominant IBS might actually be useless for *another* person with diarrhea-predominant IBS. And what do you do if you have the mixed type? The fact is *there are no universal trigger or danger foods* for people with IBS, so there is no universal IBS diet that will work for everyone. Overall, research suggests that only about one in four patients with IBS actually experience symptoms that are caused or exacerbated by things in their diet.* In the end, thinking about foods as "dangerous triggers" that can lead to IBS attacks or feeling sick is actually exactly the kind of catastrophic thinking we tried to correct in Chapter 5, "Applying the Cognitive Model to GI Symptoms."

That does not mean, however, that dietary changes can't help. Dietary changes can sometimes be *useful* in helping you minimize some of the *discomfort* associated with GI symptoms. It's just that you have to put some effort into figuring out what works and what doesn't work for *you*. There are some basic principles that are usually helpful for most people to understand and incorporate into their dietary choices. There are also some specific tricks and products that *many* (but not all!) people with IBS can benefit from. In the following pages we detail some of the most common recommendations for IBS sufferers and why they might or might not make sense for you. But the most important thing to keep in mind is that even if a particular food does cause some intestinal discomfort, it's not a disaster. That same food may well cause the same kind of intestinal discomfort to someone without IBS. If you don't panic at the first twinge, if you don't assume the worst, mild discomfort usually passes on its own.

* W. D. Heizer, S. Southern, & S. McGovern (2009). The role of diet in symptoms of irritable bowel syndrome in adults: A narrative review. *Journal of the American Dietetic Association, 109*, 1204–1214.

Remember—the whole point of this program has been to teach you not to *catastrophize* your GI symptoms. They're just annoying and uncomfortable, and occasionally inconvenient. So by all means, read on and see if any of the dietary advice listed here might be helpful. But remember that the goal is not to *eliminate* all GI sensations and symptoms from your life. That would be unrealistic. All people—normal, healthy people—have GI sensations and symptoms from time to time. It's not that big of a deal.

A SPECIAL NOTE FOR IBD PATIENTS

Much of the dietary advice in this chapter applies equally well to IBD patients when you are *not* having an active flare. However, there are certain dietary changes your doctor will advise you to make during active flares, and you should follow your doctor's advice. In particular, your doctor may recommend a "low-residue diet," in which fiber (particularly insoluble fiber) and other foods that are harder for your body to digest are restricted. This is particularly important if you have been diagnosed with intestinal strictures, in which part of the intestinal wall becomes thickened by scar tissue and the tube through which food must pass becomes too narrow and rigid. If you eat too much fiber; chunky food like nuts, beans, or popcorn; or stringy food like celery, it can actually cause a blockage at the point of the stricture. Note, however, that doctors typically recommend a low-residue/low-fiber diet for *short-term use* during disease flare-ups or following surgery to help with recovery. It is *not* a general eating plan for all people with IBD all the time.

MILK PRODUCTS

Many people with gut problems hear that avoiding milk products may be a good idea. This is based on the assumption that lactose (the sugar in milk) is "difficult to digest" for many people. You may remember from Chapter 1, "Do I Have IBS?," that lactose intolerance is frequently *misdiagnosed* as IBS because the symptoms are so similar. If your GI symptoms are really caused by lactose intolerance, then eliminating milk products that are high in lactose (or using Lactaid® products or supplements) is certainly a good idea. In fact, one study* found that 68 percent of patients with a suggested diagnosis of IBS proved to be lactose-intolerant when they were administered a hydrogen breath test. All the patients in the study were put on a lactose-free diet. Those patients who had showed no evidence of lactose malabsorption *didn't benefit from the diet at all.* But about half of the patients who were lactose-intolerant found that their symptoms *completely subsided* and another 40 percent found that their symptoms were substantially reduced. This points to the importance of a thorough diagnostic workup before you conclude that you have IBS. It also helps us understand why *some* people with "IBS" may benefit a lot from eliminating most milk products from their diet, but most people with IBS will not benefit much at all from a lactose-free diet.

WHEAT AND GLUTEN

The story with wheat- and other gluten-containing products is very similar to the story with milk products. Some people with IBS swear that eliminating gluten was the magic bullet they were looking for. But most people with IBS find that eliminating gluten does them no good whatsoever. Why? Probably because the people who benefited from eliminating gluten *really* had undiagnosed celiac disease, not IBS at all. Another research study† found that about a third of patients diagnosed

* P. Vernia, M. R. Ricciardi, C. Frandia, T. Bilotta, & G. Frieri (1995). Lactose malabsorption and irritable bowel syndrome: Effect of a long-term lactose-free diet. *Italian Journal of Gastroenterology, 27*(3), 117–121.

† U. Wahnschaffe, J. D. Schulzke, M. Zeitz, & R. Ullrich (2007). Predictors of clinical response to gluten-free diet in patients diagnosed with diarrhea-predominant irritable bowel syndrome. *Clinical Gastroenterology & Hepatology, 5*(7), 844–850.

with diarrhea-predominant IBS tested positive for the antibodies and genes that are associated with celiac disease. All the patients were put on a gluten-free diet for six months. Sixty percent of the "IBS" patients who had tested positive for the signs of celiac disease returned to *normal*, while only about 10 percent of the people who had tested negative saw any improvement in their GI symptoms at all. Again, this study points to the importance of a thorough diagnostic workup, and helps explain why some people with "IBS" may indeed benefit from eliminating gluten from their diet, but most will not.

Remember that "elimination diets" in which you try just eliminating a potential food component like lactose or gluten are *not* a good way to figure this out. You need to have the appropriate laboratory tests done to determine if you are actually either lactose-intolerant or have celiac disease and shouldn't eat gluten.

HIGH-FIBER DIETS

Few dietary recommendations get people with IBS more agitated than the simplistic recommendation to "eat more fiber." Doctors sometimes recommend increasing dietary fiber by adding wheat bran (usually in the form of cereal) or taking a fiber supplement such as Metamucil®. Some people with IBS will find that this helps, at least sometimes, particularly with constipation. Reviews of the scientific literature on the use of fiber in IBS generally conclude that fiber may have some (limited) benefit for constipation-predominant IBS, and not much benefit otherwise. But simply increasing "dietary fiber" will not be helpful to most people, and may actually make your symptoms *worse*. In fact, one study* found that 55 percent of IBS patients who had tried whole wheat and wheat bran products reported getting worse, while about 10 percent reported that

* C. Y. Francis & P. J. Whorwell (1994). Bran and the irritable bowel syndrome: Time for reappraisal. *Lancet, 344,* 39–40.

they found it helpful. Indeed, some scientific studies seem to show quite conclusively that high-fiber diets can actually *worsen* symptoms for many or even most people with IBS.

The reason for these confusing findings and conflicting advice is that there are two different *kinds* of dietary fiber. Neither kind is fully digested by the acids, enzymes, and symbiotic bacteria in our bodies, but they act very differently as they pass through our digestive system.

Insoluble Fiber

Insoluble fiber is the kind of fiber found in wheat bran, leafy green vegetables (like lettuce and spinach), and fruit and vegetable *skins*. Insoluble fiber does not dissolve in water and passes through your digestive tract largely intact. In fact, sometimes you can still recognize the food perfectly well when it comes out the other end. (For example, whole corn kernels, shreds of lettuce, or bits of tomato skin may be easy to identify in very loose stools.) In general, insoluble fiber adds *bulk* to the stools. All in all, this generally makes stools larger and softer, as long as you drink plenty of water. It also decreases "transit time" through the colon. That is, the more insoluble fiber you eat, the faster your stools will move through you. If you suffer primarily from constipation-predominant IBS, adding more insoluble fiber to your diet is probably a good idea. Just remember to drink more water, too. In general, diets relatively high in insoluble fiber promote regular bowel movements and prevent constipation. Insoluble fiber also helps your body move toxic waste through your colon in less time. This may be part of the reason that high-fiber diets are linked to a lower incidence of certain cancers.

But if you suffer primarily from diarrhea-predominant IBS, foods high in insoluble fiber should be eaten in moderation. The last thing you need is looser, more watery stools that pass through the colon more quickly! That doesn't mean you should avoid these foods altogether. Whole grains and leafy green vegetables are an important part of a healthy diet. It does mean that they should probably be eaten in small quantities at a time, combined with other foods that will cushion their effect.

Soluble Fiber

Soluble fiber does dissolve in water. It's found in bananas, carrots, oats and oat bran, rice, the flesh (but not the skins) of potatoes and sweet potatoes, and the flesh (but not the skins or seeds) of many other fruits and vegetables, including apples, avocado, berries, tomatoes, beets, squash and pumpkin, and beans and peas. While soluble fiber is not completely digested, it does break down into a gel-like substance that absorbs water as it passes through your digestive tract. Thus, soluble fiber tends to make your stools softer, but also helps them adhere and gives them shape. Soluble fiber also enhances intestinal mucus. That may sound gross, but it's a good thing. All in all, soluble fiber is helpful for *both* constipation-predominenat IBS (because it makes stool softer and more slippery) *and* diarrhea-predominant forms of IBS (because it also makes stools absorb water, hold together better, and gives them more form). Indeed, at least one recent review of the scientific literature* suggested that soluble fiber does reduce symptoms in most people with IBS, whereas insoluble fiber supplementation alone may worsen symptoms.

The best solution for most people is to combine soluble and insoluble fiber at every meal. For example, instead of having raisin bran for breakfast (where almost all the fiber is insoluble), have a bowl of oatmeal (soluble) with strawberries (soluble) and blueberries (a bit of insoluble fiber in the skin). Or better yet, make your own granola with whole rolled oats (soluble) and nuts (some soluble and some insoluble) and have it with a

* C. J. Bijkerk, J. W. Muris, J. A. Knottnerus, A. W. Hoes, N. J. deWit (2004). Systematic review: The role of different types of fibre in the treatment of irritable bowel syndrome. *Alimentary Pharmacology and Therapeutics, 19*(3), 245–251.

banana (soluble). This is a high-protein, deliciously satisfying breakfast that provides lots of heart-healthy omega-3 fats, vitamins, and minerals and should help calm a crampy gut and reduce diarrhea.

If you want to increase your consumption of soluble fiber quickly and easily, psyllium seeds may be a good source for you. Psyllium, also known as plantago or ispaghula, contains very high levels of soluble fiber. The husk or coat of the psyllium seed is about 30 percent mucilage—exactly the stuff that turns into slippery, soft, water-absorbing soluble fiber in the gut. It acts as a soothing lubricant and helps absorb excess water, making it a useful intervention for both constipation and diarrhea. Note that psyllium is the main ingredient in Metamucil, so taking Metamucil is the easiest way to add psyllium to your diet. If Metamucil aggravates your symptoms, you can try taking a smaller dose. But if it still aggravates your symptoms, psyllium is unlikely to be helpful in any form.

PROBIOTICS

Probiotics refer to live microorganisms (like bacteria) that can be ingested either in food (as in yogurt) or in a supplement pill form and are helpful to overall health. The microorganisms survive inside you once you ingest them and contribute to your health. It may seem odd to think of bacteria as something that can be good for you, but remember, our digestive system depends on millions of bacteria that *normally* inhabit our gut and help us digest our food. One of the main reasons antibiotics tend to cause diarrhea is that not only do they kill off whatever infectious agent you're taking them for (say, strep throat), but they also tend to kill off a lot of the good bacteria in your gut. Without those critters to help us break down food, it passes through relatively undigested, resulting in diarrhea. In fact, one of the most important functions of these microflora is that they ferment undigested carbohydrates and soluble fiber in the colon— thus playing a crucial role in creating the helpful, gel-like substance that binds stool, but keeps it soft. A number of recent reviews of the scientific literature on probiotics and IBS* suggest that they do seem to be helpful to most people who take them, but that it is not yet clear what the best formulations are. (People with IBD should consult with their doctors before taking a probiotic supplement. It may not be a good idea during active flare-ups, but it may be helpful at other times.)

The easiest way to consume probiotics is to eat or drink dairy products (like yogurt, buttermilk, and kefir) in which the active, live cultures are exactly the probiotic bacteria we want in our guts. Consuming probiotics in dairy products is easy, and there's some evidence that the milk product itself buffers the cultures, keeps them alive while in storage, and helps them survive the harrowing trip through the stomach acids to arrive in the gut alive and well. Even mildly lactose-intolerant people often find that they can eat yogurt without any ill effects, since the bacteria in the cultures have already broken down a good deal of the lactose.

The alternative is to purchase a probiotic supplement, usually in a pill or tablet form. Be sure to get one that has an enteric coating. Otherwise, the cultures are unlikely to survive exposure to stomach acid. The problem with probiotics is that they are considered "nutritional supplements" and are not regulated or monitored by the Food and Drug Administration. That means you don't really know what you're getting. That pill or tablet might contain exactly what the label says, or it might

---

* S. Nikfar, R. Rahimi, F. Rahimi, S. Derakhshani, & M. Abdollahi (2008). Efficacy of probiotics in irritable bowel syndrome: A meta-analysis of randomized, controlled trials. *Diseases of the Colon & Rectum, 51,* 1775–1780.

L. V. McFarland & S. Dublin (2008). Meta-analysis of probiotics for the treatment of irritable bowel syndrome. *World Journal of Gastroenterology, 14,* 2650–2661.

S. M. Wilhelm, C. M. Brubaker, E. A. Varcak, & P. B. Kale-Pradhan (2008). Effectiveness of probiotics in the treatment of irritable bowel syndrome. *Pharmacotherapy, 28,* 496–505.

R. Spiller (2008). Review article: Probiotics and prebiotics in irritable bowel syndrome. *Alimentary Pharmacology & Therapeutics, 28,* 385–396.

be nothing but dust. One brand of probiotic, Align® (which is manu-factured by Proctor and Gamble), has actually been tested in two inde-pendent clinical trials* † for people with IBS and was found to contain the actual probiotic bacterium it listed on the label (Bifidobacterium infantis) *and* was found to be helpful for IBS patients compared with placebo. Patients reported decreases in pain and bloating, and overall relief. Because it's the only brand that's been tested and proven to work, it's what I usually recommend to my patients.

PEPPERMINT

Mint has been used for millennia as a soothing digestive aid. It turns out that peppermint oil actually does relax the smooth muscles of the intestinal tract. One relatively recent, carefully controlled scientific study‡ found that 75 percent of IBS patients experienced significant symptom relief, while none of the patients receiving a placebo did. One of the most important things about this study was that the researchers tested all potential participants ahead of time for both lactose intolerance and celiac disease, and admitted only those people who tested negative for both. They also used enteric-coated capsules. This is important because straight peppermint oil hitting the stomach can cause reflux and belching that is quite unpleasant and tastes surprisingly *terrible*.

---

* L. O'Mahony, J. McCarthy, P. Kelly, et al (2005). Lactobacillus and Bifidobacterium in irritable bowel syndrome: Symptom responses and relationship to cytokine profiles. *Gastro-enterology*, *128*, 541–551.

† P. J. Whorwell, L. Altringer, J. Morel, et al (2006). Efficacy of an encapsulated probiotic Bifidobacterium infantis 35624 in women with irritable bowel syndrome. *American Journal of Gastroenterology*, *101*, 1581–1590.

‡ G. Cappello, M. Spezzaferro, L. Grossi, L. Manzoli, & L. Marzio (2007). Peppermint oil (Mintoil) in the treatment of irritable bowel syndrome: A prospective double blind placebo-controlled randomized trial. *Digestive and Liver Disease*, *39*, 530–536.

GINGER

Ginger, like mint, has been used for millennia as a digestive aid, particularly for the treatment of nausea and vomiting. While nausea is not an official symptom of IBS, according to the Rome III criteria (see page 5), some IBS patients do complain of nausea. There have been no scientific studies of the impact of ginger on IBS symptoms. However, there have been studies of the impact of ginger on nausea and vomiting associated with pregnancy and chemotherapy, and it does seem to be helpful. Moreover, studies in healthy participants suggest that ginger does have a positive impact on how the stomach processes food. Thus, there is some data to suggest that ginger (taken fresh, drunk as tea, used as a spice in food, or taken as a supplement) may indeed reduce *gastric* (or stomach) distress, nausea, and vomiting. However, since IBS typically affects the intestines, *not* the stomach, ginger is unlikely to provide substantial relief to most people with IBS.

GASSY FOODS

While there is no evidence that people with IBS actually produce *more* gas than people without IBS, there is no question that people with IBS tend to be more *bothered* by gas. Some foods are more likely to cause gas than others. Legumes (including beans, lentils, and soy), cruciferous vegetables (such as cabbage, broccoli, cauliflower, and Brussels sprouts), and onions all contain compounds that lead to the production of gas in the digestive tract as they are broken down. There are no well-controlled scientific studies of the impact on IBS symptoms of eliminating or reducing gas-producing foods. There are simple steps that can be taken to reduce the gassy by-products of some of these foods, however. Over-the-counter supplements, such as Beano® and Bean-zyme™, contain an enzyme (alpha-galactosidase) that helps break down the gas-causing compounds in legumes and cruciferous vegetables before they reach the large intestine. There *are* scientific studies* supporting the efficacy of these enzyme supplements at reducing gas and flatulence in people without IBS. So if excessive, bothersome gas, bloating, or flatulence typically follows consumption of these foods for you, it's certainly worth giving Beano or a similar product a try.

SOY PRODUCTS

As noted above, soybeans are legumes (just like black beans, kidney beans, cannellini beans, chickpeas, and lentils) and belong to the class of foods that can cause excess intestinal gas (and diarrhea) in some people. This is one of the main reasons that switching from cow's milk to soy milk–based products may do you no good at all and may actually make your symptoms worse. If you are actually lactose-intolerant, or if you just really like tofu, edamame, or soy milk and want to be able to eat soy products with no difficulty, products like Beano may help. Don't expect soy products to be the silver bullet that cures your IBS. But don't view soy as "dangerous," either. It is neither. In moderation, like just about any other food, soy products can be part of a nutritious, balanced diet for almost everyone.

FRUCTOSE, SORBITOL, AND OTHER CARBOHYDRATES

Some people with IBS swear that fructose, sorbitol, and xylitol make their symptoms worse, and that avoiding fruit and other foods with a high concentration of fructose helps enormously. It is true that some individuals

* M. DiStefano, E. Miceli, S. Gotti, A. Missanelli, S. Mazzocchi, & G. R. Corazza (2007). The effect of oral alpha-galactosidase on intestinal gas production and gas-related symptoms. *Digestive Diseases and Sciences*, *52*(1), 78–83.

(both with and without IBS) have difficulty absorbing fructose and sorbitol. (Sorbitol and xylitol are found primarily in "sugar-free" candies and gum.) When these sugar molecules are not absorbed in the small intestine, they pass on to the large intestine, where they will be fermented by bacteria. This can lead to excess gas, a change in intestinal motility, and discomfort or even diarrhea. A few studies have suggested that fructose malabsorption may be somewhat greater in IBS patients than in people without IBS, or that IBS patients may respond with more symptoms, even when hydrogen breath tests suggest similar levels of malabsorption. There have been no good controlled scientific studies yet to test whether limiting consumption of fructose (or any other carbohydrate) has any positive effect on IBS symptoms beyond a placebo effect. Moreover, it would be extremely difficult, impractical, and probably unwise to eliminate all of these foods from your diet. By all means, cut out soda and other highly processed, nutritionally empty foods that are flavored with high fructose corn syrup. Similarly, try not to consume too much sorbitol and xylitol—fake "foods" that have no nutritional value whatsoever. But eliminating whole fruits like apples, oranges, cherries, and pears will deprive you of vitamins, minerals, and a wonderful source of soluble fiber.

FODMAP FOODS

Some websites, dietitians, and gastroenterologists recommend that people with all kinds of gut problems (including IBS and IBD) follow the FODMAP diet, in which all foods high in "Fermentable Oligo-, Di- and Mono-saccaharides, and Polyols" are restricted. This diet attempts to eliminate a number of carbohydrates, which are broken down into sugars during digestion and may exacerbate gas, flatulence, cramping, and diarrhea. It's really a combination of lots of other advice—and includes eliminating dairy (lactose), wheat and rye (gluten), legumes (all beans, peas, chickpeas, and lentils), most sweeteners, and many fruits and vegetables (including some that are comfortingly high in soluble fiber, like avocado, mushrooms, and beets). In fact, the justification for these global restrictions is that restricting just one type of FODMAP food (e.g., dairy or fructose alone) doesn't work because you actually have to restrict *all* of them simultaneously. The FODMAP diet does allow *some* fruits (like bananas, citrus, and blueberries) and vegetables (including carrots, eggplant, corn, celery, and lettuce). Ironically, however, many of the vegetables tend to be relatively high in insoluble fiber, which can make diarrhea worse. There is some evidence that the FODMAP diet works for some people,* reducing gas and the volume and water content of stool, but it's hard to follow and it's hard to get decent nutrition on it. One good thing about the research on the FODMAP diet is that the scientists who study it have been careful to note that people should be tested for their ability to digest fructose and lactose with a hydrogen breath test. They note that if fructose and/or lactose absorption is efficient (and doesn't lead to lots of hydrogen gas), then there's no reason to restrict relevant foods. However, some aspects of the FODMAP diet are known to be bad for people with both IBS and acute IBD (it's relatively high in insoluble fiber and contains some high-residue foods), and it eliminates or severely limits a number of nutritious foods, many of which are high in soluble fiber. If you want to try it, you really need the guidance of a dietitian with expertise in the diet, and you need to commit to *substantial*, long-term dietary changes.

COFFEE

Coffee—even decaffeinated coffee—stimulates intestinal motility in almost everyone.† Many people with IBS choose to avoid coffee (and other

---

* P. R. Gibson & S. J. Shepherd (2009). Evidence-based dietary management of functional gastrointestinal symptoms: The FODMAP approach. *Journal of Gastroenterology and Hepatology, 25*(2), 252–258.

† S. S. Rao, K. Welcher, B. Zimmerman, & P. Stumbo (1998). Is coffee a colonic stimulant? *European Journal of Gastroenterology, 10*, 113–118.

caffeinated beverages, such as black tea and certain sodas) in hopes that it will reduce intestinal distress. There have been no good scientific studies of the impact of coffee or caffeine on IBS, however. On the other hand, eliminating these beverages from your diet is relatively easy to do, and there may be health benefits to cutting them from your diet beyond reduction in IBS symptoms. Most people find that they sleep better and enjoy more sustained energy during the day when they wean themselves off caffeine. A cup of mint or ginger tea can be a pleasant way to start the day if you crave that morning cup. On the other hand, since there is very little data suggesting that coffee exacerbates IBS symptoms, it's unlikely to be the real culprit. If you're curious about its effect on your GI symptoms, try eliminating coffee for a week or two (be prepared for some headaches the first few days if you're a real addict). See if your IBS symptoms improve. Then reintroduce coffee and watch what happens. But be careful not to catastrophize the outcome! Say you drink half a cup of coffee in the morning and fifteen minutes later you find that you experience a strong urge to defecate. Is this really so bad? Hot liquid hitting the stomach in the morning stimulates intestinal activity for most people. That could actually be a good thing! After all, many people with IBS would like to know that their bodies are predictable. You have to defecate sometime during the day. Why not first thing in the morning, halfway through your cup of coffee, but before you take your shower? On the other hand, if coffee truly makes you feel ill, then, by all means, avoid it.

MEAT AND EGGS

Red meat, dark meat from poultry, poultry skin, pork, and egg yolks are commonly perceived as dangerous "trigger" foods and are listed on many IBS-related websites as foods to avoid at all costs. However, *there is no data from any study suggesting that this is true.* You may choose to avoid different types of meat for any number of reasons, including on religious, environmental, ecological, economic, or moral grounds. There are dozens of well-designed studies suggesting that diets *relatively* low in red meat and saturated fat contribute to an overall healthy lifestyle and reduce your long-term risk of heart disease and some cancers. But this has nothing to do with IBS or digestive health. The main problems with meat in America are twofold. First, we tend to eat too much of it in a single "serving." Second, too many of the animals we eat are raised in inhumane ways and fed unnatural diets of grain (as opposed to grass) that cause the *animals* all sorts of digestive problems and infections, and lead directly to the overuse of antibiotics on feedlots. Ironically, it is these *animals* that suffer from horrible gastrointestinal problems, and their fat is far worse for our cardiovascular health than the fat of grass-fed, organically raised animals. But there is no evidence that eating meat from these animals causes gastrointestinal problems in humans.

Egg yolks have been demonized by a number of groups, primarily because they contain high levels of cholesterol. They are also typically listed in the "must avoid" column on many lists of IBS trigger foods because of their high fat content. But egg yolks also contain high levels of vitamins E, A, and D; folate; riboflavin; and omega-3 fatty acids, all of which are essential and contribute substantially to health in many ways. If you throw out the yolk, you throw out most of the nutritional value in an egg beyond the pure protein. By all means, spend a few extra dollars a week and purchase organic eggs laid by cage-free hens. Their eggs tend to contain even more of the healthy fats and vitamins we need, and you can feel good about supporting ethical and ecologically sound farming practices. But don't throw out those yolks! Eat whole eggs, as nature intended.

FRIED FOOD AND FATTY FOOD

Eating a diet relatively low in fried food is probably a good idea for everyone. A huge platter of barbecued spareribs or fried chicken, French fries or greasy biscuits, and coleslaw or corn on the cob slathered in butter may or may not send you running to the bathroom, but it won't be good for you, no matter how you look at it. Eat fried and fatty foods occasionally and in small portions to save your waistline and your heart. This is good dietary advice for all of us. But don't expect that limiting these foods will magically relieve your IBS.

SPICY FOODS

Spice can refer to any number of substances that are used to flavor food, making it more pungent, aromatic, or tasty. Cinnamon and nutmeg are both spices that do not seem to contribute to IBS symptoms at all. Curry—the classic Indian combination used to spice many foods—includes ginger and turmeric, which may actually reduce gastrointestinal distress for some people. Although some people with IBS prefer to avoid garlic, another pungent spice, there is little evidence that it serves as a trigger food for many individuals with IBS. On the other hand, capsaicin, which is the chemical that makes chili peppers "hot," may in fact contribute somewhat to abdominal pain in people with IBS. One recent study[*] did find evidence of increased sensitivity and density in the sigmoid colon of nerves that respond to capsaicin. In addition, the density of those nerve cells was correlated or related to abdominal pain in individuals with IBS. So there is a chance that reducing or avoiding exposure to "hot" or "picante" foods might be a good idea. You yourself can be the best judge. As with coffee, it might be worth doing a behavioral experiment—avoiding those foods for several weeks, and then intentionally eating a spicy meal to see what happens. As always, the key is to avoid catastrophizing the results of eating those foods. You may be a bit uncomfortable, which is annoying. But it does not need to be a catastrophe.

[*] A. Akbar, Y. Yiangou, P. Facer, J. R. F. Walters, P. Anand, & S. Ghosh (2008). Increased capsaicin receptor TRPV1-expressing sensory fibres in irritable bowel syndrome and their correlation with abdominal pain. *Gut, 57,* 923–929.

SUMMARY

In summary, there may be some foods that don't agree with you, at least some of the time, and there may be some strategies that will help keep your gut functioning smoothly, efficiently, and regularly. But there are also a lot of myths out there, and following all the advice there is on diet and IBS will lead to an unnecessarily limited diet and lots of unnecessary anxiety about "dangerous" trigger foods. To recap:

- Limiting dairy products is unlikely to help, unless you're lactose-intolerant.

- Limiting wheat and other sources of gluten is unlikely to help, unless you have celiac disease.

- Elimination diets are *not* an appropriate way to diagnose lactose intolerance or gluten sensitivity. You need to have laboratory testing (a hydrogen breath test, and blood work to identify celiac antibodies) to know for sure.

- Increasing insoluble fiber will be helpful only if you have constipation-predominant IBS. Be sure you drink plenty of water, along with consuming the extra fiber. If you have diarrhea-predominant or mixed-type IBS, simply increasing insoluble fiber is likely to make you feel worse.

- Consuming more *soluble* fiber is probably a good idea no matter what kind of gut problems you have, since soluble fiber tends to help with both constipation and diarrhea. Eating a balanced diet in which you combine soluble and moderate amounts of insoluble fiber at every meal is probably the best strategy.

- Adding probiotics to your diet, either in the form of yogurt or in nutritional supplements like Align, may indeed help and certainly won't hurt.

- Peppermint oil supplements may help relax the smooth muscles in your colon.

- Ginger can reduce nausea but is unlikely to help with most IBS symptoms.

- Foods that tend to produce gas (like beans, soy foods, and broccoli) are perfectly safe to eat, but many people (including people without IBS) find that Beano reduces uncomfortable gas and flatulence.

- While it is *possible* that fructose malabsorption plays a small role for a few people with IBS, eliminating fruit from your diet is impractical and unwise. By all means, however, cut out sodas and other processed foods that contain lots of high fructose corn syrup, and limit your exposure to "fake" sugars like sorbitol and xylitol.

- The FODMAP diet, which tries to eliminate a wide range of foods containing carbohydrates that may be poorly absorbed (including lactose and fructose), is a very complex, highly restrictive diet that requires the guidance of a registered dietitian to follow safely. It involves eliminating a wide range of foods, including dairy, gluten, legumes, many fruits and vegetables, and sweeteners. It may work to reduce symptoms in some individuals with IBS and IBD, but such a restrictive diet can compromise nutrition and should not be attempted on your own.

- Coffee stimulates colonic motility in just about everyone. If you find, after testing it systematically, that it worsens your cramping and diarrhea, don't drink it. But if you love that morning cup, then enjoy knowing that you're likely to poop every morning at a predictable time.

- There is no evidence that meat or egg yolks contribute to intestinal distress in people with IBS. Treating them as "dangerous" just contributes to the perception that something is horribly wrong with you and the world of food is an unsafe place. Eat meat in moderation. If you can, buy grass-fed, organic beef and organic cage-free chicken. Buy organic eggs, but don't throw out the yolks! You deprive yourself of most of the wonderful nutrition nature put into those perfect little packages.

- Very greasy, fried food isn't good for anyone. Eat it infrequently and only in small quantities.

- Many savory, tasty dishes are just fine to eat. There is a little bit of data suggesting that chili peppers may aggravate intestinal cramping and pain in people with IBS. Test this systematically in yourself and see if it holds true for you.

- If you have an IBD, follow your doctor's advice about specific dietary restrictions during active flares. If you're unsure as to why your doctor is making a particular recommendation, ask!

In the end, your goal should be to find a balanced, tasty, and nutritious diet for yourself that is relatively high in fruits and vegetables (peeled if you need to), legumes (taken with Beano), nuts and some whole grains (with a bit more emphasis on oats and rice than wheat and corn), and with lots of heart-healthy fats (from nuts and olive oil). Your diet may include a reasonable portion of animal protein, which can include dairy, whole eggs, and meat of all kinds (unless you prefer a vegetarian diet for other reasons), *in moderation*. Your diet should generally be low in processed foods, caffeine, and nutritionally "empty" calories from soda and candy. Avoid "fake" foods, like olestra and artificial sweeteners. Do this and it will be good for your heart, your brain, and your waistline. It may or may not ultimately eliminate your GI symptoms, but it will definitely be good for you.

Chapter Nine

SUMMARY, REVIEW, AND FINAL THOUGHTS

I started this book by reviewing other conditions that have symptoms that are very similar to IBS. Current medical practice is to diagnose IBS on the basis of a review of symptoms, an abdominal exam, some simple blood work to rule out anemia and infection/inflammation, and a stool test. Much of the research literature on diet and IBS suggests that it's very important to conclusively rule out lactose intolerance and celiac disease as well, and your doctor should be open to discussing these possibilities with you. If you don't have "alarm" symptoms (like anemia, fever, bloody stool, or abdominal pain that awakens you at night), then you can probably forgo more invasive testing like colonoscopy, unless you are over age fifty. However, if you're having any other problems (like vitamin deficiencies), or there are signs of inflammation in some of your tests (like the fecal calprotectin test), or if you just aren't comfortable with the IBS diagnosis, then you should certainly consider asking your doctor for a colonoscopy, an MRE, and/or a capsule endoscopy to rule out the inflammatory bowel diseases Crohn's and ulcerative colitis. Getting a positive diagnosis and ruling out the other obvious potential causes of symptoms is the first step to getting your IBS under control.

Unfortunately, it *is* possible to have both an inflammatory bowel disease and symptoms that are consistent with a functional disorder like IBS, especially if you continue to have significant GI symptoms when the IBD is in remission. So even if you have a history of Crohn's disease or ulcerative colitis, the information and skills in this book should still be useful to you. IBD and IBS may share some underlying biology (like inflammation and disruption in the normal ecosystem of intestinal bacteria). Stress has a physical effect on the gut, no matter what else is going on biologically, so reducing stress should help reduce your GI symptoms, no matter what your diagnosis is. And gut problems are stressful, no matter what caused them to begin with.

In the second chapter, "What's Causing My Gut Symptoms?," I reviewed what's known about IBS. Remember that IBS is caused by a combination of biology, psychology, and environmental stressors. Every one of us has some system in our body that reacts to stress. Some of us get back pain or spasms in our neck and shoulders, some of us get terrible headaches, some of us grind our teeth or bite our nails, or break out in hives. Others are particularly vulnerable to effects of stress on the GI system. Your gut is your "weak link" because you're prone to visceral hypersensitivity and abnormal intestinal motility. Your enteric nervous system is a little bit overreactive and responds too strongly to interactions with the sympathetic nervous system. This means your gut will react a lot to psychological and environmental stressors. You may have a chronic, low-grade inflammatory stress response going on. The symbiotic intestinal bacteria that help all of us digest food and modulate the inflammatory response in the gut may be compromised somehow in your system. In addition, you may have developed catastrophic beliefs about your GI symptoms themselves that contribute to your level of stress and make your gut problems much more disabling. Assuming that you've had appropriate medical workups that have ruled out other potential problems (like lactose intolerance, celiac disease, active Crohn's disease, and ulcerative colitis), you can rest assured that the symptoms of IBS are *annoying* but not *harmful*. You are *not sick*, and thinking of yourself as sick probably isn't terribly helpful.

I then strongly suggested that you regularly practice one or more relaxation techniques. Since the physiological arousal associated with stress can actually make GI symptoms worse, reducing physiological arousal can be very helpful. Deep breathing, done correctly, is a particularly useful exercise because it can be done anywhere, any time, without anyone noticing. Even if imagery and/or progressive muscle relaxation work well for you—and it's great if they do—I suggest you keep working on deep breathing until you can feel yourself relax after two or three deep breaths.

I then introduced the basic cognitive model, which suggests that our reactions to situations—our feelings, physical symptoms, and behaviors—are the result of our *beliefs* about situations, rather than the situations themselves. Oftentimes, people with gut problems have lots of negative beliefs. Some of those negative beliefs are general ones that occur across lots of different types of situations. Other negative beliefs relate directly to GI symptoms themselves. GI-related beliefs tend to fall into two categories: beliefs about how intolerable symptoms are and beliefs about the social and occupational implications of symptoms. Since beliefs can be right or wrong, it makes a lot of sense to identify our negative thoughts and try to look at them a bit more objectively. This includes trying to generate *benign alternatives* to our negative beliefs, and then considering the evidence we have for and against each set of beliefs. *Behavioral experiments,* which can provide us with relevant data we wouldn't normally have access to, can be very helpful in challenging deeply held or upsetting beliefs.

The best way to learn these techniques is to practice them, usually by actually writing up a worksheet, after the fact, when you have a little more distance and perspective, and can take the time to think things through. Eventually, though, it would be much more useful to you if you could begin to identify and question your negative automatic thoughts *in the moment*, while stressful things are actually occurring. Now, obviously, you can't just whip out a worksheet during a meeting or while you're on a date or talking to your kid's teacher. That *would* be weird! But the nice thing about this is that the more you practice coming up with benign alternatives to negative thoughts, the more automatic *positive* thoughts will start to become. Most people find that they don't need to keep using the actual worksheets for very long. They begin to catch the negative thoughts right as they crop up. Eventually, you start to question those thoughts the instant they occur to you. People report thoughts like this:

"Oh, geez, he must think I'm an idiot. My gut hurts—this is going to be awful. Wait a second—I actually have a point here—and my gut is roiling because I hate conflict. But if I stick to my guns, he'll listen. My gut is a little crampy, but that can't stop me from finishing this . . ."

When I see people in my private practice, they often tell me that at first the positive thoughts actually sound like they're in my voice! People will tell me they hear me saying to them, "Now wait a second . . . Is that the best way of thinking about it?" We usually have a good laugh about it—they can't get rid of me! In time, though, as people get better at it, the positive thoughts start to be in their own voice. By the end of treatment, they're often not even conscious of the process of questioning negative thoughts and replacing them with more reasonable ones. It just starts to happen automatically. Negative thoughts still occur to them from time to time, but these thoughts have much less power and feel much less compelling and upsetting. So people are able to dismiss them much more quickly.

Because this book doesn't take long to work through, you may not find that this happens to you right away. It may take weeks or even several more months. Don't give up! Keep practicing things after the fact, and eventually you'll start to be able to do it in the moment, when stressful things are actually happening. Even if you can't do it in the moment, lots of times we ruminate and obsess about upsetting things after the fact. If these skills help you do less of that, then that's a good thing, too.

The final piece of any treatment program for gut-related problems involves identifying situations that people have been *avoiding*, including examples of *subtle avoidance,* and then using the techniques of exposure therapy to try to overcome that avoidance. Avoidance is often the most life-damaging aspect of GI problems—more than any physical discomfort or inconvenience. People stop traveling, stop eating out, stop going to parties, stop shopping, sometimes even stop working and socializing. If this is you, you've allowed your gut problems to cheat you out of work, love, and play—the three most essential components of any healthy, happy life. It's essential that you *reclaim your life*. Don't allow negative, catastrophic thoughts that may not even be true to limit what you do or where you go. Use the techniques outlined in Chapter 7, "Eliminating Avoidance"— reread that chapter if you need to—to help you design an individualized program that will get you back to all aspects of living.

As a final exercise, it might be interesting to revisit the questionnaires you completed at the beginning of the book—the ones that measured GI symptom severity, visceral sensitivity, catastrophic beliefs about GI symptoms, and IBS-related quality of life. You can find them again now in Appendices B, C, D, and E. Try filling them out again with a different color pen. Most people will find that their scores have changed a lot. If that's you, congratulations! You are well on your way to reclaiming your life from IBS.

WHEN TO ASK FOR PROFESSIONAL HELP

I really hope this book has been helpful to you and that your IBS isn't bothering you nearly as much as it was before you worked through this program. However, it's important to acknowledge that not everyone will be able to get everything they need from a self-help book. Sometimes problems are complicated, long-standing, or just entrenched. Many people with IBS also face other challenges. People with IBS are more likely than people without IBS to struggle with depression and anxiety. Self-help is great, but there's nothing quite like having a dedicated, supportive, and highly skilled professional working with you to understand and address the places where you're getting stuck. If you feel like you're still struggling—if you're still unhappy, unmotivated, exhausted, overwhelmed, or worried a lot of the time, or if your gut symptoms are still out of control and impairing your life, then it may be time to think about seeking professional help from a psychiatrist or a psychologist with a background in cognitive behavioral therapy.

Almost all therapists (including social workers, counselors, psychologists, and psychiatrists) are warm, caring, supportive people. They wouldn't have gone into the field if they weren't. But not all therapists are trained the same way. Some therapists may be very kind and personally insightful, but may not have the specific skills they need to help with particular problems. Cognitive-behavioral therapy (CBT) is one of the few types of therapy that has been *proven* to work for a wide range of problems, including depression, panic disorder, social anxiety disorder, generalized anxiety disorder, obsessive-compulsive disorder, and a range of chronic health-related issues, including IBS. A good way to find out if there is a CBT therapist close to you is to visit the Find a Therapist webpages at one of the professional organizations that specializes in promoting good science in the diagnosis and treatment of behavioral health concerns. These organizations include the Association of Behavioral and Cognitive Therapies (ABCT.org), the Anxiety and Depression Association of America (ADAA.org), and the Academy of Cognitive Therapy (academyofct.org). All three websites allow you to search geographically to find therapists in your area. If you can't find someone in your area, try calling your insurance provider and asking specifically if the company has any therapists in its network who are trained in CBT.

One final option to consider is medication—not antidiarrheals like Imodium or Lomotil!—but medications that work in the brain to help modulate the neurochemicals involved in depression, anxiety, and pain. You will typically need to see a psychiatrist for this (although some internists, general practitioners, and gastroenterologists might feel comfortable and confident prescribing these particular medicines for the treatment of IBS). The only medications with a good scientific track record in helping people with IBS are several different groups of medicines collectively known as "antidepressants." The name is misleading because many medicines can be used to treat different things. For example, aspirin can be used to reduce fever. It can also be used to reduce the pain of migraine headaches and the very different pain of sore muscles. It can *also* be used to reduce the risk of heart attack and stroke. So if we called aspirin an "antifever" drug, it really wouldn't tell the whole story and it would be confusing. You might very well want to take aspirin when you didn't have a fever at all. The same thing is true of the so-called antidepressants. These medicines can affect a number of different processes, including digestion and pain. Which exact medicine you might consider trying depends a lot on your primary symptoms.

There are three basic classes of antidepressant medicines that might make sense to consider. The oldest group is known as the *tricyclic family (TCAs)*. They mostly affect a neurotransmitter in the brain called norepinephrine. They've been around for decades and they're all available generically (so they're less expensive). TCAs include:

> Amitriptyline (Elavil®)
>
> Imipramine (Tofranil®)
>
> Desipramine (Norpramin®)
>
> Nortriptyline (Pamelor®)

TCAs tend to cause *constipation* as a side effect. This might be pretty inconvenient for someone who was taking the medicine for depression, but for someone with diarrhea-predominant IBS (especially with urgency), this can be a terrific outcome that normalizes bowel movements and helps break the IBS cycle.

The next family of medicines is the *selective serotonin reuptake inhibitors (SSRIs)*. The first, and most famous, SSRI was Prozac® (Fluoxetine), but there are many others, including:

> Sertraline (Zoloft®)
>
> Citalopram (Celexa®)
>
> Escitalopram (Lexapro®)
>
> Paroxetine (Paxil®)

SSRIs tend to cause diarrhea, at least initially, when people start taking them, so these medicines may be better for people who have constipation as part of their IBS. They can help a *lot* with stress reactivity, depression, and anxiety, though, so if the SSRI-driven exacerbation of diarrhea resolves relatively quickly, they can be pretty helpful.

The final and newest family of medicines are those called *serotonin-norepinephrine reuptake inhibitors (SNRIs)*. They include:

> Venlafaxine (Effexor®)
> Duloxetine (Cymbalta®)
> Desvenlafaxine (Pristiq®)
> Milnacipran (Savella®)

Interestingly, the SNRIs have been found to be quite helpful in treating chronic pain conditions, like fibromyalgia and peripheral neuropathy, and some preliminary studies have suggested they help with visceral (gut) pain as well. Because they affect both norepinephrine (which can make you constipated) *and* serotonin (which can give you diarrhea), the GI side effects tend to cancel each other out and you mostly get the benefits of the anti-pain, anti-inflammatory (and antidepressant) effects, so the SNRIs can be helpful for people with all types of IBS.

It's important to understand that *none* of these medicines are addictive and you won't become dependent on them. There *are* medicines that are addictive and cause physiological dependence and tolerance—these include the stimulants (like Ritalin® [methylphenidate] and Adderall® [amphetamine and dextroamphetamine]) and the antianxiety drugs from the family called benzodiazepines (like Xanax® [alprazolam], Valium® [diazepam], and Klonopin® [clonazepam]). Interestingly, *all* of these drugs are also sold illegally as "street drugs" because you can get high by taking them. *No one would ever sell Elavil, Prozac, or Effexor illegally—because no one would buy it!* They don't make you high. They don't even elevate your mood. If you're depressed, they take at *least* two weeks (and often up to six weeks) to kick in and start making you feel better. They don't change your personality—although they can make negative, catastrophic thoughts less intense, and they might make it easier to learn and use the cognitive-therapy skills taught in this book. The relief you get from them isn't fake—it's just *you* at your best. If IBS patients find that a medicine is helping, most will elect to stay on it for at least six months to a year. Many people can go off at that point. Especially if you've worked through a program like this, you may well find that you don't need it anymore. On the other hand, if your IBS symptoms do come back (or you find that you feel more depressed or anxious, or just that it's taking too much *energy* to manage your thoughts and feelings), then it might make a lot of sense to stay on the medication longer. This isn't a personal failure or a defeat. It's just smart, proactive management of a set of complex medical conditions.

FINAL THOUGHTS

There is considerable evidence that many, many people can work through a self-help program like this one on their own and get a *great deal* of benefit from it. In fact, this very workbook was tested in a randomized, controlled trial* (the gold standard in science for showing that a treatment actually works), and the people who completed it typically experienced a lot of relief. Their visceral sensitivity went down, and so did their catastrophic thoughts about their GI symptoms. They reported experiencing fewer IBS symptoms and being much less bothered by them when they did experience them. Most importantly, their quality of life improved. They stopped avoiding things and felt like their IBS symptoms had much less impact on them. Hopefully, you will find that working through this book has been similarly beneficial for you. So keep breathing! Consider things objectively. Catch your negative automatic stressful thoughts and correct them. Don't let IBS cheat you out of work, love, and play. *Reclaim your life!*

* M. G. Hunt, E. Ertel, J. A. Coello, & L. Rodriguez (2014). Empirical support for a self-help treatment for IBS. *Cognitive Therapy and Research, 39*(2), DOI 10.1007/s10608-014-9647-3.

FINAL THOUGHT RECORD

SITUATION	THOUGHTS

FEELINGS	ALTERNATIVES & EVIDENCE

FINAL THOUGHT RECORD

SITUATION	THOUGHTS

FEELINGS	ALTERNATIVES & EVIDENCE

FINAL THOUGHT RECORD

SITUATION	THOUGHTS

FEELINGS	ALTERNATIVES & EVIDENCE

FINAL THOUGHT RECORD

SITUATION	THOUGHTS

FEELINGS	ALTERNATIVES & EVIDENCE

ACKNOWLEDGMENTS

I would be remiss if I did not acknowledge the contributions of several generations of undergraduate students at the University of Pennsylvania who have helped me develop and test the treatment in this book. Samantha Moshier and Marina Milonova worked with me on my very first study with IBS patients, helping to establish the theory of GI-specific catastrophic cognitions. They encouraged me to develop a treatment for IBS based on that theory and helped me test it in a randomized, controlled trial (RCT) that was administered via the Internet and included limited therapist feedback to patients. Jordan Coello and Amy Kranzler encouraged me to develop a short self-report questionnaire for measuring GI-specific catastrophizing. Jordan, and later Elisabeth (Lissy) Ertel and Lauren Rodriguez, helped me validate that new measure. Together with Amber Calloway, they also encouraged me to turn the short, modular Internet treatment protocol into a full-fledged, stand-alone self-help book. Jordan read several early versions of the manuscript, helping to make sure it struck the right tone and used the right voice, and helped get the RCT to test it off the ground. Lissy and Lauren then shepherded the full-fledged clinical trial through the last stages of data collection and follow-up. I am very grateful to all of them for their invaluable contribution to this work. I truly could not have done it without them. I'm also very proud of all of them for pursuing careers in psychology or medicine. I think they're all superstars and we're lucky that the next generation of clinical scientists includes such bright and talented young people.

I'm also grateful to my colleague Dianne Chambless for encouraging me to test my new self-help book in a true RCT before seeking to publish it. Dianne has always been a key voice in the field of clinical psychology, demanding that therapeutic treatments have empirical, scientific support. I'm glad I followed her advice and I'm very proud of the fact that I published the scientific paper proving that this book was helpful to people before I approached the good folks at Sterling.

I owe a tremendous debt to the many talented and phenomenally skillful clinicians who taught me how to be a therapist. I am deeply grateful to Robert DeRubeis, Cory Newman, Maryanne Layden, Vic Malatesta, Peter AuBuchon, Judy Salzberg, Ruth Greenberg, Judith Coché, and, of course, the always astonishing, creative, and brilliant Dr. Aaron T. Beck. I am incredibly lucky to have learned from the best, and I hope I channel their collective wisdom, insight, and good humor in everything I do with patients.

Thanks to my agent, Marilyn Allen, who helped me make the leap from publishing in scientific journals to reaching a larger audience of real people in the real world.

Thanks to Kate Zimmermann at Sterling, who respected my voice and has helped relieve much of my anxiety about saber-toothed editors.

Thanks to my parents, Bob Hunt and Irene Winter, who still model for me the joys of an intellectual life and how to balance work, love, and play; who encouraged me and believed in me; and who celebrate my successes with genuine pride.

Thanks to my wonderful kids, Ian, Noah, and Anna Rose, who have put up with my twice-weekly "late nights" for years so I could see my evening patients, analyze data, write papers with students, and finish this book. I have so enjoyed watching all three of them grow into such amazingly successful, smart, talented, loving, and interesting young people.

Finally, thanks to my beloved husband, Garth Isaak, without whom life would simply not be possible. He is my partner in every way that matters and every way I need. I still can't believe how lucky I am.

APPENDIX A

ROME III CRITERIA QUESTIONNAIRE

You probably have IBS if you pick a **bold** answer for all of the following questions:

1. In the last three months, how often did you have discomfort or pain anywhere in your abdomen?

    0—Never → Skip remaining questions

    1—Less than one day a month

    2—One day a month

    3—Two to three days a month

    4—One day a week

    5—More than one day a week

    6—Every day

2. For women: Did this discomfort or pain occur only during your menstrual bleeding and not at other times?

    0—No

    1—Yes

    2—Does not apply because I had the change in life (menopause) or I am male.

3. Have you had this discomfort or pain six months or longer?

    0—No

    1—Yes

4. How often did this discomfort or pain get better or stop after you had a bowel movement?

> 0—Never or rarely
> **1—Sometimes**
> **2—Often**
> **3—Most of the time**
> **4—Always**

You need a **bold** *response to either question 5 or question 6.*

5. When this discomfort or pain started, did you have more frequent bowel movements?

> 0—Never or rarely
> **1—Sometimes**
> **2—Often**
> **3—Most of the time**
> **4—Always**

6. When this discomfort or pain started, did you have less frequent bowel movements?

> 0—Never or rarely
> **1—Sometimes**
> **2—Often**
> **3—Most of the time**
> **4—Always**

You need a **bold** *response to either question 7 or question 8.*

7. When this discomfort or pain started, were your stools (bowel movements) looser?

> 0—Never or rarely
> **1—Sometimes**
> **2—Often**
> **3—Most of the time**
> **4—Always**

8. When this discomfort or pain started, how often did you have harder stools?

> 0—Never or rarely
>
> **1—Sometimes**
>
> **2—Often**
>
> **3—Most of the time**
>
> **4—Always**

Questions 9 and 10 help you determine what subtype of IBS you have.

If you pick a **bold** answer for question 9 and pick 0 for question 10, you have constipation-predominant IBS. If you pick 0 for question 9 and pick a **bold** answer for question 10, you have diarrhea-predominant IBS. If you pick a **bold** answer for *both* questions, you have the mixed subtype.

9. In the last three months, how often did you have hard or lumpy stools?

> 0—Never or rarely
>
> **1—Sometimes** (About 25% of the time)
>
> **2—Often** (About 50% of the time)
>
> **3—Most of the time** (About 75% of the time)
>
> **4—Always** (100% of the time)

10. In the last three months, how often did you have loose, mushy, or watery stools?

> 0—Never or rarely
>
> **1—Sometimes** (About 25% of the time)
>
> **2—Often** (About 50% of the time)
>
> **3—Most of the time** (About 75% of the time)
>
> **4—Always** (100% of the time)

APPENDIX B

GASTROINTESTINAL SYMPTOM RATING SCALE (GSRS)

Please rate your degree of discomfort with each of the following symptoms over the last week.

	Not at all	Mi
1. Have you been bothered by abdominal pain during the past week?	0	
2. Have you been bothered by pain or discomfort in your abdomen, relieved by a bowel action during the past week?	0	
3. Have you been bothered by a feeling of bloating during the past week?	0	
4. Have you been bothered by passing gas during the past week?	0	
5. Have you been bothered by constipation (problems emptying the bowel) during the past week?	0	
6. Have you been bothered by diarrhea (frequent bowel movements) during the past week?	0	

Mild	Moderate	Somewhat Severe	Severe	Very Severe
2	3	4	5	6
2	3	4	5	6
2	3	4	5	6
2	3	4	5	6
2	3	4	5	6
2	3	4	5	6

	Not at all	M
7. Have you been bothered by loose bowel movements during the past week?	0	
8. Have you been bothered by hard stools during the past week?	0	
9. Have you been bothered by an urgent need to have a bowel movement (need to go to the toilet urgently to empty the bowel) during the past week?	0	
10. Have you been bothered by a feeling that your bowel was not completely emptied after having a bowel movement during the past week?	0	
11. Have you been bothered by feeling full shortly after you have started a meal during the past week?	0	
12. Have you been bothered by feeling full even long after you have stopped eating during the past week?	0	
13. Have you been bothered by visible swelling of your abdomen during the past week?	0	

Mild	Moderate	Somewhat Severe	Severe	Very Severe
2	3	4	5	6
2	3	4	5	6
2	3	4	5	6
2	3	4	5	6
2	3	4	5	6
2	3	4	5	6
2	3	4	5	6

To score the GSRS, just add up the numbers you circled.

My Score _____

Mild: 0–19   Moderate: 20–39   Severe: 40–78

APPENDIX C

IBS QUALITY OF LIFE QUESTIONNAIRE (IBS-QOL)

Please rate how much you feel each of the following statements applies to you:

1. I feel helpless because of my bowel problems.

2. I am embarrassed by the smell caused by my bowel problems.

3. I am bothered by how much time I spend on the toilet.

4. I feel vulnerable to other illnesses because of my bowel problems.

5. I feel fat because of my bowel problems.

6. I feel like I'm losing control of my life because of my bowel problems.

7. I feel my life is less enjoyable because of my bowel problems.

8. I feel uncomfortable when I talk about my bowel problems.

9. I feel depressed about my bowel problems.

10. I feel isolated from others because of my bowel problems.

Not At All	A Little	Moderately	Quite a Bit	A Great Deal
0	1	2	3	4
0	1	2	3	4
0	1	2	3	4
0	1	2	3	4
0	1	2	3	4
0	1	2	3	4
0	1	2	3	4
0	1	2	3	4
0	1	2	3	4
0	1	2	3	4

11. I have to watch the amount of food I eat because of my bowel problems.

12. Because of my bowel problems, sexual activity is difficult for me.

13. I feel angry that I have bowel problems.

14. I feel like I irritate others because of my bowel problems.

15. I worry that my bowel problems will get worse.

16. I feel irritable because of my bowel problems.

17. I worry that people will think I exaggerate my bowel problems.

18. I feel I get less done because of my bowel problems.

19. I have to avoid stressful situations because of my bowel problems.

20. My bowel problems reduce my sexual desire.

21. My bowel problems limit what I can wear.

22. I have to avoid strenuous activity because of my bowel problems.

23. I have to watch the kind of food I eat because of my bowel problems.

24. Because of my bowel problems, I have difficulty being around people I don' know well.

Not At All	A Little	Moderately	Quite a Bit	A Great Deal
0	1	2	3	4
0	1	2	3	4
0	1	2	3	4
0	1	2	3	4
0	1	2	3	4
0	1	2	3	4
0	1	2	3	4
0	1	2	3	4
0	1	2	3	4
0	1	2	3	4
0	1	2	3	4
0	1	2	3	4
0	1	2	3	4
0	1	2	3	4

25. I feel sluggish because of my bowel problems.

26. I feel unclean because of my bowel problems.

27. Long trips are difficult for me because of my bowel problems.

28. I feel frustrated that I cannot eat when I want because of my bowel problem

29. It is important to be near a toilet because of my bowel problems.

30. My life revolves around my bowel problems.

31. I worry about losing control of my bowels.

32. I fear that I won't be able to have a bowel movement.

33. My bowel problems are affecting my closest relationships.

34. I feel that no one understands my bowel problems.

To score the IBS-QOL, first add up the numbers you circled:

Total of numbers circled _____

ot At All	A Little	Moderately	Quite a Bit	A Great Deal
0	1	2	3	4
0	1	2	3	4
0	1	2	3	4
0	1	2	3	4
0	1	2	3	4
0	1	2	3	4
0	1	2	3	4
0	1	2	3	4
0	1	2	3	4
0	1	2	3	4

Now divide your total by 136: _____ / 136 = _____

Now multiply that number by 100 to get your final score:

_____ x 100 = _____

Minimal or Mild: 0–31   Moderate: 32–66   Severe: 67–100

APPENDIX D
VISCERAL SENSITIVITY INDEX (VSI)

Below are statements that describe how some people respond to symptoms or discomfort in their belly or lower abdomen. These may include pain, diarrhea, constipation, bloating, or a sense of urgency. Please answer *how strongly you agree or disagree* with each of these statements, as they relate to you. Answer all of the statements as honestly and thoughtfully as you can.

1. I worry that whenever I eat during the day, bloating and distension in my be will get worse.

2. I get anxious when I go to a new restaurant.

3. I often worry about problems in my belly.

4. I have a difficult time enjoying myself because I cannot get my mind off of discomfort in my belly.

5. I often fear that I won't be able to have a normal bowel movement.

6. Because of fear of developing abdominal discomfort, I seldom try new foods

7. No matter what I eat, I will probably feel uncomfortable.

rongly isagree	Moderately Disagree	Mildly Disagree	Mildly Agree	Moderately Agree	Strongly Agree
0	1	2	3	4	5
0	1	2	3	4	5
0	1	2	3	4	5
0	1	2	3	4	5
0	1	2	3	4	5
0	1	2	3	4	5
0	1	2	3	4	5

8. As soon as I feel abdominal discomfort, I begin to worry and feel anxious.

9. When I enter a place I haven't been before, one of the first things I do is to lo[?] for a bathroom.

10. I am constantly aware of the feelings I have in my belly.

11. I often feel discomfort in my belly could be a sign of a serious illness.

12. As soon as I awake, I worry that I will have discomfort in my belly during the d[?]

13. When I feel discomfort in my belly, it frightens me.

14. In stressful situations, my belly bothers me a lot.

15. I constantly think about what is happening inside my belly.

ongly sagree	Moderately Disagree	Mildly Disagree	Mildly Agree	Moderately Agree	Strongly Agree
0	1	2	3	4	5
0	1	2	3	4	5
0	1	2	3	4	5
0	1	2	3	4	5
0	1	2	3	4	5
0	1	2	3	4	5
0	1	2	3	4	5
0	1	2	3	4	5

To score the VSI, just add up the numbers you circled.

My Score _____

Mild: 0–10   Moderate: 11–30   Severe: 31–75

APPENDIX E

GI COGNITIONS QUESTIONNAIRE (GI-COG)

Please rate the degree to which you believe each of the following statements:

1. If I feel the urge to defecate and cannot find a bathroom right away, I won't be able to hold it and I'll be incontinent.

2. The thought of fecal incontinence is terrifying. If it happened, I would never get over the humiliation.

3. If I fart, people around me will be disgusted.

4. If I don't drink or eat with other people, they will think I'm antisocial and no fun.

5. If I have to get up and leave an event, meeting, or social gathering to go to the bathroom, people will think there's something wrong with me.

6. If I have to interrupt a meeting or presentation at work to go to the bathroom, will be awful, and people will think I'm incompetent or unreliable.

7. If I have to stop or leave to find a bathroom during an outing or trip, my friends and family will be frustrated and annoyed with me.

Hardly at All	A Little Bit	Moderately	A Fair Bit	Very Much
0	1	2	3	4
0	1	2	3	4
0	1	2	3	4
0	1	2	3	4
0	1	2	3	4
0	1	2	3	4
0	1	2	3	4

8. If I told my coworkers about my gut problems, they wouldn't understand and would think I was weak or gross.

9. When I feel my GI symptoms acting up, I'm afraid the pain will be excruciat and intolerable.

10. When my gut acts up, I have to cancel my plans and miss out on important parts of life.

11. If I'm experiencing a gut attack and feeling sick, I can't enjoy or pay attentio anything else.

12. It is unfair and horrible that I have to have these awful symptoms.

13. If people knew about my gut problems, they would think about me negativel

14. If I leave the house without my emergency medicine(s) (e.g., Imodium®, Lomotil®, Pepto-Bismol®, Gas-X®, Tums®), it could lead to disaster.

15. Having to deal with gut problems is incredibly embarrassing.

16. If people knew what my life was really like, they would think I was crazy.

Hardly at All	A Little Bit	Moderately	A Fair Bit	Very Much
0	1	2	3	4
0	1	2	3	4
0	1	2	3	4
0	1	2	3	4
0	1	2	3	4
0	1	2	3	4
0	1	2	3	4
0	1	2	3	4
0	1	2	3	4

To score the GI-COG, just add up the numbers you circled.

My Score _____

Mild: 0–19   Moderate: 20–39   Severe: 40–64

APPENDIX F

DAILY SYMPTOM LOG

Date	Symptoms	Severity (0 not at all–5 extrem
	Abdominal pain	
	Change in frequency of defecation	
	Change in stool consistency	
	Gassy	
	Urgency to defecate	
	Straining to defecate	
	Unable to empty bowel	

Possible Stressors

APPENDIX G

FOOD SOURCES OF SOLUBLE FIBER

Food Source	Soluble Fiber (g)	Total Fiber (g)
CEREAL GRAINS (½ cup [119 ml] cooked)		
Barley	1	4
Oatmeal	1	2
Oat Bran	1	3
Psyllium Seeds, 1 Tbsp	5	6
FRUITS		
Apple	1	4
Banana	1	3
Blackberries (½ cup [119 ml])	1	4
Orange	2	2–3
Grapefruit	2	2–3
Nectarine	1	2
Peach	1	2

Food Source	Soluble Fiber (g)	Total Fiber (g)
Pear	2	4
Plum	1	1.5
Prunes (¼ cup [59 ml])	1.5	3
LEGUMES (½ cup [119 ml] cooked)		
Black Beans	2	5.5
Kidney Beans	3	6
Lima Beans	3.5	6.5
Navy Beans	2	6
Northern Beans	1.5	5.5
Pinto Beans	2	7
Lentils	1	8
Chickpeas	1	6
Black-eyed Peas	1	5.5
VEGETABLES (½ cup [119 ml] cooked)		
Broccoli	1	1.5
Brussels Sprouts	3	4.5
Carrots	1	2.5

INDEX